How To Cut
Your Medical Bills

How To Cut
Your Medical Bills

Art Ulene, MD
Val Ulene, MD

Ulysses Press

1994

Published by: Ulysses Press
P.O. Box 3440
Berkeley, CA 94703-3440

Library of Congress Catalog Card Number 93-60475

ISBN 0-915233-95-9

Printed in the USA by The George Banta Company

10 9 8 7 6 5 4 3 2 1

Cover Design: Bonnie Smetts
Background photography: Will Crocker/Image Bank
Back cover photo: David Quinney
Color Separation: Twin Age Limited, Hong Kong

Distributed in the United States by Publishers Group West.

CONTENTS

INTRODUCTION

How much are you paying for your family's health care? No matter what part of the country you live in, no matter how large or small your family, you probably feel you're paying too much.

You need to look no further than your own checkbook to get a painfully clear picture of the high cost of modern medicine. According to one estimate, health care for the average American carried a price tag of $3,380 in 1993. As a nation, we collectively spent $903 billion to treat our illnesses and keep ourselves well. No wonder there is so much talk—from the Oval Office to the kitchen tables of middle America—that the system is out of control and in need of emergency care. Without immediate intervention, the delivery of medical services will bankrupt the nation and its people.

WHY SUCH A HIGH PRICE TAG?

There are many reasons for the spiraling costs of medicine. Perhaps the most obvious is the high price tag that comes with cutting-edge technology. Whereas physicians of an earlier era relied on tongue depressors and tender loving care to nurse their patients back to health, today we depend—indeed, we insist—upon the latest gadgets science has to offer. While it is impossible not to be impressed with CT scans and magnetic resonance images that provide detailed pictures of the inner workings of the human body, with each new technological breakthrough, the cost of medicine spirals further out of control. Add to that the unconscionable price gouging done by some doctors, hospitals and insurance companies, the unnecessary tests and surgeries that are performed without justification, and the fraudulent claims made by some consumers—no wonder the system is in a state of fiscal hemorrhage.

As this book goes to press, politicians and other interested parties are finally making efforts to stop the bleeding with something more substantial than verbal Band-Aids and makeshift legislative tourniquets. In the meantime, many people have simply been priced out of the marketplace, denied the best that medicine has to offer and left to fend for themselves to keep their families healthy. Even amid this crisis, however, some hospitals continue to encourage doctors to overutilize expensive diagnostic equipment to bring in added revenue, and many doctors still order questionable tests for no reason other than to practice "defensive medicine" that supposedly protects them against malpractice suits.

While modern medicine has made many extraordinary breakthroughs, there is still something nostalgically appealing about simpler times when doctors made house calls and provided care that nearly everyone could afford. And although we can't turn back the clock, there is a growing demand for a return to both sensible medicine and common sense.

TAKING BACK CONTROL

We've written this book for and about *you*, the medical consumer. We believe you can rise above the chaos in the medical marketplace, and ensure that your family is well protected and cared for, no matter what paths the politicians take in the years ahead.

Frankly, it is tempting to presume that the Clinton Administration and Congress will resolve the health care emergency for us. But that's a risky assumption. Keep in mind that even in the best-case scenario, the Clinton Administration plans to phase in its health care reforms over a period of five or more years. In all likelihood, by the year 2000, the changes will still be evolving, and the goals for a fairer, fully accessible system will not yet be achieved.

Thus, we urge you *not* to become complacent. In fact, even if you already have good health insurance, you still need to remain alert to what lies ahead. Why? Because under the Clinton plan, you could actually end up with *worse* coverage than you presently have.

Just consider this fact: In the fall of 1993, as President Clinton unveiled his blueprint for a revitalized health care system, he proposed a "core package" of benefits for all Americans--a commendable goal, but one which may *take away* protection from those who are presently well insured. That means even if you now have comprehensive coverage, you may not have it in the future—or you'll have to pay much more out-of-pocket for the same level of protection. In other words, health care may well persist as a critical issue for you in the years ahead.

Now more than ever, we think you need to sharpen your skills and find ways to make the best use of your health care dollar. And that's what this book can help you do. It can empower you and everyone else who reads it. As simplistic as it may sound, the American people can accomplish more in reducing health care costs than any govern-ment master plan, no matter how well conceived. For example, what if we all became cost conscious enough to save just $10 a year in med-ical expenses? Multiply that $10 by 250 million Americans, and that's a collective savings of $2.5 *billion* dollars, without relying on politi-cians, doctors or hospital administrators. Yes, each of us can make a significant difference in how much the country spends on health care.

ENSURING QUALITY

There's another important reason to curtail our spending for medical care—and it may surprise some people: As our health care expendi-tures decline, the quality of care is likely to increase. That's right, increase! Of course, most people believe that the opposite is true, con-vinced that the *more* they spend, the better their care will be.

But studies show something quite different. If you undergo more tests and are given more medications than you need, your risk of complications, side effects, and inaccurate test results will multiply. Good care equates with getting only what you need, and getting it done right the first time. The fact is, the better your medical care, the less it will usually cost! Keep in mind that you really can get too much of a "good" thing. Quality care sometimes means *less* care, including knowing when to stay away from the doctor's office.

Of course, there are times when you absolutely *should* see a doctor. When you're really sick, seek medical attention quickly. If you experi-ence severe and persistent chest pain, for instance, you could be having a heart attack, and rapid treatment could save your life! But if you've got minor symptoms like a runny nose, don't rush to the doctor's office at the first sneeze. Be patient. An expensive doctor's visit may not be beneficial to either your health or your pocketbook.

MAKING THE RIGHT CHOICES

The best way to minimize your medical expenses is to keep yourself healthy, and thus stay out of the system as much as possible. Our own negative health habits are responsible for up to 70 percent of all hospitalizations. In fact, studies show that under the age of 65, our lifestyle is the single greatest factor affecting our chances of survival. By contrast, medical care is responsible for only 10 percent of this equation. Throughout this book, we'll emphasize prevention and show you other ways you can cut health care costs while improving your health.

GETTING STARTED . . .

We believe this is a book that you can refer to again and again in the months and years ahead. We'll provide you with guidelines on making the best decisions regarding your health care in the present and the future—helping to ensure that you obtain good medical and hospital treatment when you need it, and *only* when you need it. We'll also show you how to get that care in a cost-effective manner, without sacrificing quality. We'll describe how to choose the right doctor, how to select the best insurance plan, how to cut costs for medical tests and hospitalization.

To repeat, this book is about personal empowerment. Knowledge is power, and the information here will help you get excellent care at competitive prices. It can turn you into a smart medical consumer. And when that happens, your health—and your pocketbook—will reap the benefits.

HOW TO SAVE MONEY ON HEALTH INSURANCE

As health care costs continue to soar, it's more important than ever to have good—and reasonably priced—medical insurance. Unfortunately, hospital and doctor bills aren't the only things on the rise. The premiums on health insurance are climbing so high and so fast that a lot of folks are being priced right out of the marketplace. Even so, if you know your way through the health insurance maze, you can avoid most of the quagmires and quicksand, and get yourself and your family the coverage you need.

As this book went to press, the Clinton Administration was just introducing its health care reform package to Congress. Many months of debate are expected before a vote is reached on Capitol Hill. Although the ultimate fate of this health care package is unknown, one thing is certain: Any legislation passed by Congress in 1994 or beyond will not be fully implemented for many years, probably not before the end of this decade. Until then, and perhaps even beyond, you will still need to make important decisions about health insurance for you and your family. For that reason, read this chapter carefully and use its information wisely, no matter how health care reform evolves in the years ahead.

Why Health Insurance?

No matter what your health status, your age or your income—and no matter how expensive health insurance may seem—you really can't afford to do without it.

The purpose of health insurance is simple: To provide you and your family with protection against the potentially bankrupting cost of illness. If health insurance were cheap and if it paid all your medical bills, there really would be no need for you to educate yourself about the ins and outs of buying coverage. You'd simply write a modest check for your insurance each month, see your doctor when necessary, and never give the cost much thought. But at least for now, that isn't the way the health insurance game is played. Unless you're among the wealthiest few, you probably can't afford enough insurance to cover all your medical expenses. Consequently, you need to start making some informed decisions to find the right balance in the insurance you select, protecting yourself against medical catastrophes while avoiding financial ruin just to pay for your coverage.

A NECESSITY, NOT A LUXURY

Everyone needs health insurance. No matter what your health status, your age or your income—and no matter how expensive health insurance may seem—you really can't afford to do without it. A single uninsured catastrophic illness could wipe out your savings and leave you and your family digging out of debt for years. Frankly, it's not worth the risk.

Just imagine trying to pay for some of today's expensive medical procedures out of your own pocket. Even relatively common surgeries carry stunning price tags. The average cost of a coronary artery bypass operation, for example, is about $49,000. Faced with a potential medical bill that steep, nearly everyone needs some medical insurance to fall back on.

Let's face it: None of us knows what the future holds. You and your family may have been fortunate enough to enjoy good health for years. But you have no way of predicting if, in the months ahead, your spouse might have a heart attack, your son might break a leg during football practice, or your daughter might be involved in a serious bicycle accident. Health insurance is necessary, although you can make it less of a burden by choosing your coverage carefully.

Health insurance provides another major dividend, too. Recent studies show that if you have health coverage, you'll actually receive better medical treatment. When a doctor or hospital knows that you have the means to pay your bill, you'll get a higher standard of care. It may not be fair, but it's a fact of life. For example, one study showed that among uninsured patients, bypass surgery is performed 29 percent less often than in insured patients. According to a 1989 study reported in the *New England Journal of Medicine*, newborns from uninsured families have a 31 percent greater risk of having adverse experiences in the hospital. Overall, the risk of dying in the hospital is significantly greater for the uninsured! It may not sound right, but many doctors and other health care providers make treatment decisions based on who can pay—and who can't.

Group Insurance: The Best Buy?

There's no such thing as a bargain anymore when it comes to health insurance. Even so, some alternatives are better than others. If you're able to get your coverage through your workplace, you may have a huge advantage over people who need to go hunting for protection on their own, in terms of both cost and benefits. Actually, most Americans—nearly 71 million of them—get their health insurance at their place of employment. If it's available to you there, that's where you should start looking.

The Sooner the Better

Keep in mind that as you get older, your chances of developing illnesses will increase. Depending on the nature of those illnesses, you could become ineligible for the comprehensive coverage you can purchase today. You're probably never going to be healthier than you are now, so don't take unnecessary risks with either your health or your pocketbook. The sooner you buy insurance, the better.

> *Most Americans—nearly 71 million of them—get their health insurance at their place of employment.*

In recent years, however, a crisis in work-based insurance has been gradually evolving. A growing number of businesses are being severely squeezed by the financial crunch of skyrocketing insurance costs, and have been forced to rethink what they can offer their workers. In 1992, the price tag for providing health insurance for the average American employee was over $3,900. That's a significant expense, and for some companies, it represents as much as 20 percent of their total payroll costs. No wonder so many employers have started to scream for help, looking to the government or just about anyone else for a solution—while recognizing that there are no easy answers.

Corporate America has responded to this health insurance crisis in a number of ways. Many companies have been forced to pass along more of the costs of coverage to their employees. Others have cut benefits. If you get your health insurance at work, you may have noticed significant changes occurring in your own health package or you may see them soon. For example:

- Your protection may not be as comprehensive as in the past. Coverage for visits to dentists or orthodontists may have been eliminated. Or there may have been cuts in insurance for mental health services or for pregnancy and childbirth.

- You may be responsible for paying a greater portion of your health care costs than ever before. While your employer might have once paid for your health insurance in full, you may now be required to make a contribution to the premium, as well, perhaps as a deduction from your paycheck each week.

- Coverage for your family members may no longer be an employer-paid benefit. You might have to pay for their insurance, in part or in full.

- Your deductible may be higher now than in the past. Thus, you will have to pay more of your medical bills out-of-pocket before the insurance company begins to cover them.

- Your employer might be encouraging you to participate in a so-called "managed care" program, such as an HMO (health maintenance organization), which can be less costly to employer and employee, but which might limit your choice of doctors.

- You may need to get permission from the insurance company before you undergo nonemergency surgery or most other major medical treatment. The insurer may have limitations on how much it will pay for these procedures, and how long your hospital stay should be for a particular medical condition.

- To save money, your employer may switch health insurance carriers, moving to a company that offers less expensive rates,

The Perils of Employer Self-Insurance

Because health care has become so expensive, many financially strapped employers are looking seriously at any option that might reduce their costs. Some have turned to self-insurance.

Under this plan, the employer does not contract with an insurance company to provide health care benefits for its workers. Instead, all the premium payments are placed in a pool, and when a claim needs to be paid, funds are withdrawn and money is sent to the doctor or hospital.

At first glance, this approach might sound appealing. But beware: It's fraught with potential problems, particularly for the employees whose health care rests in the balance. By self-insuring, a company is exempt from any state requirements for supplying employees with minimum benefits. Consequently, inadequate coverage is sometimes the rule rather than the exception, something you would know only if you had carefully read your policy.

There's another big risk with self-insuring: If one employee has a catastrophic illness, that employee's high medical bills might wipe out the entire pool of reserves, leaving everyone in the company without coverage. For this reason, some observers have described self-insurance as a disaster waiting to happen.

Nevertheless, there are ways for a good self-insurance program to protect itself from that kind of nightmare. The employer can purchase independent catastrophic coverage for employees and their families, so that everyone is protected if a major illness occurs.

but that might not handle claims as quickly or as fairly as you're used to.

Yes, times are changing. And as they do, you may feel confused and vulnerable—since most of these changes are out of your control. In the past, you may have believed you "had it made" because of your employer-provided coverage. But not anymore. Instead, you may actually find yourself searching elsewhere for your health insurance—perhaps for a policy to supplement your company coverage, but in many cases for basic protection, too. On occasion, employers have been willing to give their workers a "rebate" equal to the cost of their workplace-based health insurance, and let employees use those funds to buy coverage on their own. This has allowed people to shop around for insurance, seeking a policy that best meets their needs.

SHOULD YOU "JUMP SHIP"?

It all depends. If you currently have group coverage, don't be too quick to give it up. It still may be the best option in a complex market. Yes, your group policy may be getting more expensive, but so are all other kinds of coverage. Also, insurance companies still tend to give discounts to employers who can bring them a large volume of business and perhaps handle some of the paperwork, thus reducing the insurance company's administrative costs. You also were probably able to get your group coverage without having to take a physical exam. That's a big advantage if you've been plagued by a chronic illness.

Still, if you're not happy with your group health insurance and the direction in which it's headed—or if you're unemployed, concerned about being laid off, or worried about your company going out of business—you might want to begin investigating the alternatives. For instance, you may find that group insurance is available through a trade or professional association to which you belong. It might be cheaper or more comprehensive than the coverage you presently have. If you're an alumnus of a college, you might be eligible for its health insurance at group rates. Or perhaps better group insurance is available at your spouse's workplace. Explore your options. You might find that you can get more for your dollar elsewhere.

Instead of group coverage, you can also purchase an individual insurance policy. While group insurance is usually (but not always) less expensive, you might actually save money in the long run by declining the group coverage and tailoring an individual medical policy to your family's unique needs. Or if your group policy is lacking in certain areas—perhaps the coverage for your dependents is not as good as you would like, or there is no coverage at all for prescription drugs or maternity care—you might want some supplemental individual insurance to fill in the gaps.

Spend an evening carefully studying the protection you currently have. While some states require that insurers offer a minimum benefits package, others do not, so it's important to know the extent of your coverage, and look elsewhere for supplemental insurance if

How Good Is Your Coverage?

A good health insurance policy should provide coverage (or partial coverage) in most or all of the following areas:

- Inpatient hospital services (including semiprivate room charges, emergency room care, intensive care unit, etc.)
- Surgical services (including surgeon's and anesthesiologist's fees, use of the operating room, outpatient or "ambulatory" surgery)
- Ambulance services
- Doctor's visits (office and hospital)
- Coverage for children (up to at least age 19, or if they're full-time students, age 23)
- Newborn services
- Maternity care, including cesarean sections
- Preventive care/checkups
- Prescription medication
- Laboratory tests and x-rays
- Home health care
- Physical therapy
- Psychiatric and mental health services
- Drug and alcohol abuse treatment
- Hospice care

there are serious shortcomings in your group protection. First, check with your employer, and find out if there are ways to improve the benefits package of the company's group plan. You might be surprised to find that for a few extra dollars a month, you can bring your policy up to a more comfortable level. If there's not a way to strengthen it, however, you're not necessarily stuck with what you have; you may decide to decline the coverage and customize an individual policy that's right for you. If you do choose alternative coverage, make sure it's in force before dropping your other insurance so you don't get caught without coverage. And check to be sure you can rejoin your company's policy at a later date should something happen to your alternative coverage. If you can't, you might not want to take the risk of switching.

The rest of this chapter will help you make wise health-insurance choices. While much of the information will be particularly useful when shopping for an individual policy, the same guidelines can help you better understand, utilize and perhaps choose among the alternatives available in your group coverage. Wherever you ultimately get your health care protection—whether it's group or individual coverage—many of the same recommendations will apply.

Your Health Insurance Options

For many years, nearly all health insurance policies provided so-called "fee-for-service" coverage. It's probably the kind of protection with which you're most familiar. With this kind of health insurance, you are billed for the medical services you receive—whether from a doctor, a hospital, or a laboratory—and your insurance carrier pays most or all of the bill.

But fee-for-service plans (also sometimes called "indemnity" plans) no longer have the health insurance playing field to themselves. In recent years, an alphabet soup of other options—involving HMOs, PPOs and IPAs—have gained popularity. Whether you receive your coverage through a group or individual policy, you'll probably find some new alternatives available to you. Let's take a closer look at the options:

FEE-FOR-SERVICE

This traditional form of health coverage generally allows you more flexibility than you'd receive with other types of health insurance. For instance, if you like the idea of having no restrictions on your selection of doctors and hospitals, then look for a fee-for-service plan (although in recent years, even some of these policies have begun placing some limitations on your choices).

With fee-for-service coverage, your doctor bills you (or your insurance company) for your care, and the insurer commonly pays 80 percent of it, leaving you responsible for the remaining 20 percent. This type of arrangement is called co-insurance, meaning that both you and the insurance company share in the payment of your medical bills. The policy probably also includes a provision for a deductible, which is the amount of health care costs you are responsible for in full each year before the insurance company begins making payments. If your deductible is $200, for example, you will need to pay the first $200 in medical bills you accumulate that year, after which the insurance company begins contributing its 80 percent (or other stipulated percentage) of all subsequent costs. Deductibles are sometimes as low as $100, and can be as high as $5,000.

When you're considering buying fee-for-service protection (or any other type of health insurance, for that matter), be sure you understand fully what is—and isn't—covered in the policy. We can't repeat this enough: Make sure you read the policy's fine print, not just the attractive advertising and sales brochures. Few (if any) policies cover everything, and you need to find out now what might be excluded. Don't wait until you need it, only to find out you don't have it. Look over the services listed in the box on page 11, good insurance should cover most or all of them.

You might find that policies differ in the way their benefits are defined—that is, one policy might cover hospitalization 365 days a year; another might cover a maximum of only 30 days per "benefit period" (meaning per illness or injury), and may require a waiting period of perhaps 90 to 180 days before a new benefit period begins. One policy might pay for the full cost of a semiprivate hospital room; another might impose a limit (say, $350 or $400 per day).

> *Make sure you read the policy's fine print, not just the attractive advertising and sales brochures.*

What about preventive health care? Are you covered for routine physical exams? For mammograms? For Pap tests? If the policy includes dental care, does it cover orthodontia, too? Check the scope of the maternity insurance in the policy—since premiums are often less expensive if maternity care is deleted, consider purchasing a policy without it if you have no plans for having children. After all, it doesn't make sense to pay for protection that you will never use. Other types of services (e.g., dental care, psychiatric care) may be nice to have, but if they add considerably to the cost of the insurance, you might decide they're not worth it.

Once you've read through the policy, ask the insurance representative to clarify any areas you're unsure about. Request more than an explanation—ask to see it in writing in the policy. If it's not spelled out in the policy, you're not covered for it, no matter what verbal promises you've been given.

MANAGED CARE

In recent years, managed care programs have emerged as alternatives to fee-for-service medicine. As studies show them to be an effective means for reducing health care costs—without sacrificing the capability of providing excellent standards of care—both employers and individuals are turning to them in massive numbers. If there isn't already an HMO or a PPO in your life, there could be one in your future. In fact, many states now require employers with 25 or more employees to offer a managed care program as a health care option for their workers.

Managed care is essentially a prepaid health program that combines health insurance with a delivery system for medical care. Each month, you and/or your employer pay a monthly premium, and in return you'll receive most or all of the medical care you require. If you stay well and don't utilize the system much, the managed care system will come out ahead; but if you and your family have numerous or serious illnesses, you'll get the care you need, no matter how much the costs exceed your monthly premium.

This means there's an incentive built into managed care systems for doctors to control costs and keep you healthy. For this reason, preventive medicine is often emphasized. That's quite a bit different from fee-for-service plans, which may encourage overuse of the system; after all, the more services that are ordered or delivered, the greater the payment to doctors and hospitals.

Not everyone likes managed care, however. The most common complaint: "When I joined a managed care program, I gave up my freedom in choosing doctors and hospitals." Yes, this may seem like a sacrifice to you, but it's being made in exchange for lower costs. For many managed care subscribers, the financial benefit makes the tradeoff worthwhile.

Your employer may give you a choice between several types of managed care systems. HMOs (health maintenance organizations) and PPOs (preferred provider organizations) are the most popular, and warrant a closer look.

HMOS

Like other managed care systems, HMOs provide health services for a fixed, prepaid premium. A good HMO will cover your doctor's office visits, hospital services, outpatient surgery, maternity care, laboratory tests, prescription drugs, physical exams, and most of the other services listed in the box on page 11. In the majority of these plans, there are no deductibles, and the co-insurance payments are usually small. For example, in addition to the monthly premium, you will probably pay a small charge (perhaps $5) for each office visit, and another $2 to $3 for each prescription drug; compared to a fee-for-service plan, your out-of-pocket expenses are minimal.

The biggest and best-known HMO is Kaiser-Permanente, which was launched during World War II by businessman Henry J. Kaiser to provide health care to employees at his plants and shipyards. Today, it provides medical services for 6.6 million people (not just Kaiser workers) and employs 9,000 physicians. These doctors and Kaiser's other health care professionals work directly for the HMO. Unlike a fee-for-service plan, subscribers to the Kaiser program are covered for care only from those doctors and hospitals that are a part of the Kaiser empire.

For many consumers, the restrictions on doctor choice are a tough adjustment to make. After all, if you've had the same trusted family doctor for years, it's not surprising that you don't want to change. Even so, many HMO subscribers have found that the picture isn't as grim as it sounds. In most HMOs, there are many physicians to choose from, and if you're dissatisfied with one, you can generally switch to another within the system. Some HMOs have even contracted with physicians in private practice to care for some of their patients—a system called an IPA, or individual practice association. (These doctors also treat their own fee-paying patients, and so do not have exclusive contracts with the HMO.)

If you have a catastrophic illness, the HMO won't let you seek out doctors at the Mayo Clinic or the Texas Heart Institute—at least not if you want to be covered by the plan. However, every HMO has its own specialists on staff who can handle just about any major health concern, from open heart surgery to cancer treatment. On occasion, if a particular type of care or procedure is available only from an outside specialist or facility, the HMO will pay for that service if it approves that care in advance.

What are some of the other complaints of HMO members? Much of the criticism of HMOs is aimed at the inevitable bureaucracy of a large organization. There might be delays in getting appointments for routine care, including nonemergency operations. There may be long waits in reception rooms. HMO clinics and hospitals also may not be conveniently located. Subscriber costs of HMOs are rising, too, as all medical care has become both more sophisticated and more expensive.

HMOs—The Future?

In 1970, only about 3.6 million Americans were members of HMOs; by 1990, that figure had soared to more than 35 million, spread out over 550 different HMOs. HMOs are now a major player in the health care marketplace. If cost pressures continue, you can expect them to wield even more influence in the years ahead, and gain loyalty among even more of the population.

Nevertheless, we're not trying to paint too grim a picture of HMOs. After all, waits and delays are often part of fee-for-service medicine, too. And if you ask HMO members if, overall, they are pleased with the quality of their care, many will proba- bly give you a positive response. One

> *Add the substantial cost sav- ings available through HMOs, and it's no wonder that they have won millions of converts in recent years.*

survey by National Research Corporation of 90,000 consumers found greater patient satisfaction with HMOs than with more traditional health care delivery. Numerous other studies have reached similar con- clusions about quality of care: They show that when it comes to serious diseases like cancer, cardiovascular disease, and diabetes, HMOs offer patients medical care that is just as good as (and sometimes better than) that received by non-HMO patients. Add the substantial cost savings available through HMOs, and it's no wonder that they have won millions of converts in recent years.

What's the bottom line? There are both good and bad fee-for-service and HMO plans. One approach isn't inherently better than the other, although an HMO is more likely to help you control your medical costs. The questions in the box on pages 18-19 can help you analyze the quality of care you might receive at a particular HMO.

WHAT ABOUT PPOS?

Just when you thought you had finally made sense out of HMOs, IPAs, and fee-for-service medicine, there's still another popular option that might be available to you: PPOs, or preferred provider organizations. As insurance companies look for ways to keep the costs of health care under control, one of their increasingly successful alternatives is the PPO: a network of doctors and hospitals ("pre- ferred providers") who have agreed to provide care to patients at a negotiated rate, as a way of drawing patients to their own offices. PPOs may contract with several insurance companies and employers to provide health care services for group policy members.

If you use a PPO, you'll probably receive a booklet listing the pre- ferred providers in your community. In most cases, your employer will give you the option of using these preferred providers, or going

to any doctor that you want. However, because PPOs agree in advance
to deliver care at a reduced fee, some of the savings will be passed on
to you to encourage you to use them. Perhaps you'll be offered a
smaller deductible—maybe $150 instead of $250—or no deductible at
all when using the PPO. Or your co-payment will be reduced (per-

Before You Sign on the HMO's Dotted Line...

Prior to joining an HMO, you should ask the following questions:

- Is the HMO "federally qualified"? To achieve this designation,
  an HMO must meet federal standards in providing certain basic
  services, including physicians' care, inpatient and outpatient
  hospital services, laboratory and x-ray procedures, short-term
  mental health services, and an array of preventive health care
  (e.g., vaccinations, well-child care, family planning services).

- How many years has the HMO been in operation? How big is
  its enrollment? An HMO with a track record of at least three
  years and a large roster of enrollees (25,000 or more patients)
  should make you feel more comfortable about placing your
  family's well-being in its hands.

- How are appointments made and what is the waiting time? If
  you become really ill, you shouldn't have to wait long to see a
  doctor. A child's ear infection or strep throat often requires a
  physician's prompt attention. Can the HMO accommodate
  these kinds of needs?

- What are the background and qualifications of the HMO's doctors? Find out if all doctors are board-certified, meaning that
  they have passed competency exams. In particular, ask about
  the primary care physician you'll be seeing: Where did he go to
  medical school? Where did she do her residency and specialty
  training?

- Can you see a physician outside the HMO? Some HMOs contract with doctors in private practice to see some of their
  patients in their own offices. In other HMOs, you can only use
  their full-time staff physicians, who generally work only out
  of the HMOs' own offices.

haps you'll pay 10 percent of doctor's fees in the PPO, and 25 to 30 percent for non-PPO physicians.

In a sense, PPOs might offer the best of both worlds. On the one hand, if you're willing to give up some freedom of choice in your

---

- What specialists are available to treat a particular chronic illness? If you have heart disease, diabetes, arthritis or another serious, chronic condition, ask in advance about what specialized care the HMO can provide. Keep in mind that if you go outside the HMO system, you will probably have to pay for that care out of your own pocket.

- How extensive are the plan's nursing home benefits? If you are elderly and the HMO only provides for limited nursing home use, you might want to look at other options.

- What happens if I get sick out of town? While most HMOs will cover the cost of emergency services if you need immediate medical attention far away from the plan's nearest facility, they generally won't pay for more routine office visits. If you spend a lot of time at a vacation home in another part of the state or country, find out if the HMO has doctors or facilities nearby, or if it has reciprocity agreements with HMOs in that area.

- What do the HMO's patient satisfaction surveys show? Most HMOs conduct patient satisfaction polls of their members once or twice a year. Ask to see copies of the results, and inquire about any concerns that were raised by patients, and whether the plan has made efforts to correct these problems. Also inquire about the physician turnover rate; if it's more than three to five percent per year, it could be a sign of doctor dissatisfaction and possible troubles in the internal workings of the system.

- What type of grievance procedures are available for HMO subscribers? If you ever have a complaint, either about the availability of services or their quality, it's good to know there is a system in place to deal with complaints fairly and quickly.

doctors, you'll reap the financial benefits. On the other, you can still see any doctor you choose who is unaffiliated with the PPO, although you'll be asked to pay a larger portion of the bill. That's quite different from an HMO, which generally won't pay any portion of your medical bills if you go outside the system.

How to Choose Your Insurance

There are a lot of alternatives available for health insurance coverage, each of them seemingly more attractive than the next, thanks to flashy TV ads, celebrity endorsements, and fast-talking insurance agents. It's up to you to select the plan that best fits your needs. Following are some guidelines that can help you sort out the facts and choose the insurance plan that's right for you.

HOW STRONG IS THE INSURANCE COMPANY?

When buying insurance, be sure that the company you're considering is strong and reliable. "Great" coverage at a low price isn't worth much if the company files for bankruptcy when you're seeking reimbursement for a claim.

There are a number of companies that rate insurance carriers, examining their financial statements, evaluating their service records, and giving them a "grade" that can range from A+ to F. For instance, A.M. Best publishes its ratings in a book entitled *Best's Insurance Reports—Life/Health*, available in most public libraries. Similar types of ratings are issued by Standard and Poor's, Moody's, and Duff and Phelps.

Another source for information on an insurance company's financial stability is Weiss Research. Weiss will prepare a report for you on any of 1,900 insurance firms. Their fees vary depending on the type of report you'd like. For $15, you can get a verbal evaluation over the phone. A one-page brief is available for $25, while for $45, you can obtain a more in-depth report. For more information, contact Weiss Research at 800-289-9222.

Your state insurance department can also provide useful information. This government agency helps regulate the insurance industry, and handles consumer complaints about particular companies and agencies. In Chapter 10 of this book (page 269), we have included a list of state insurance departments throughout the country. Contact the agency in your state and ask about the level of public complaints for particular insurance firms. A file full of customer gripes is a sign to look for coverage elsewhere.

> *When buying insurance, be sure that the company you're considering is strong and reliable.*

COMPARING POLICIES

When you buy health insurance, you want to get the most for your money, so when choosing a policy, cost will be important. With group insurance, here's what you need to keep in mind:

- With a fee-for-service plan, you may have to pay at least a portion of the monthly fee (premium), unless you're lucky enough to have an employer who pays for all of it. You will also be responsible for a deductible and co-payments.

- With a managed care program, your employer will probably pay the entire premium, leaving you with only a small co-payment each time you use services.

As important as cost is, it's just one of the factors you must weigh. Don't overlook the comprehensiveness of the coverage. No matter what type of policy you're leaning toward—group or individual—carefully study the benefits being offered. All policies look alike when you hold them in your hand, but they can vary dramatically in what they offer.

Check to see if a policy excludes coverage for certain illnesses called pre-existing conditions. If you join a health insurance plan and have been treated for heart disease or cancer, for example, in recent months or years, you may find that your policy excludes coverage for your particular condition—for a "waiting period" of at least six months or a year, but sometimes longer, depending on what state you live in. Be wary of policies that exclude coverage for pre-existing conditions; they may not be worth much if there's no coverage for the conditions for which you're most likely to be treated.

> *Be wary of policies that exclude coverage for pre-existing conditions; they may not be worth much if there's no coverage for the conditions for which you're most likely to be treated.*

When shopping for insurance, never lose sight of your own family's needs. If you have children, look for coverage that includes pediatric care, beginning at the moment of birth. If you or other family members use a lot of prescription drugs, make sure you have coverage in this area. If it appears that you are being shortchanged on the particular benefits you know that you and your family will need, look elsewhere.

At the same time, don't overbuy. It's foolish to buy more protection than you actually need. If you and your spouse are senior citizens, you don't need to pay extra for maternity benefits or well-baby care. If you're a healthy young person, you may not need comprehensive prescription drug coverage until later in life when you're more likely to use it. Health insurance is expensive enough; don't inflate the cost even more by paying for something that may be unnecessary.

READ THE FINE PRINT

Although the language in many insurance policies has been simplified and is easier to read than it was a few years ago, these documents are still essentially legal agreements, and the fine print can be confusing. Nevertheless, don't let yourself become intimidated. If you're getting lost in the legalese and jargon, and there's something you don't understand, ask your company's benefit office or an insurance company representative for help.

As you review the policy, the fine print should state that your coverage is renewable. If your health takes a turn for the worse, your insurance company would love nothing better than to drop you as a customer. Make sure it can't. Look for the "guaranteed renewal" clause. Yes, your insurance company does have a right to raise your premiums as you grow older, but with a renewable policy, those rates can rise only at the same pace as policies of other people your age. With a renewable plan, the insurer also won't be able to arbitrarily cancel your protection when the term of your policy expires just because you've made a lot of claims in recent months.

WHAT'S THE RIGHT DEDUCTIBLE FOR YOU?

As mentioned earlier, the deductible is the amount of medical costs you pay each year before your insurance policy kicks in and begins covering your health care expenses. Deductibles can run from $100 to $5,000. There are even "first dollar" policies, which begin covering you with no deductible at all.

Which deductible makes the most sense? Your first instinct might be to choose the lowest deductible available. That decision would seem to make sense, since the sooner your insurance company begins paying benefits, the better.

That logic, however, ignores one important fact: The lower your deductible, the higher your premium will be. You're going to be charged much higher rates for a $100 deductible than for a $500 deductible, simply because the insurance company is responsible for paying your medical bills at a much earlier point. The best rule of thumb is to take as large a deductible as you feel you can afford (especially if you are in excellent health and the likelihood of using your insurance to pay a claim is low). Yes, those initial medical costs will have to come out of your own pocket, but if you stay well, that's money you may never have to spend. At the same time, you'll keep your fixed payments (your monthly premium) relatively low.

Make sure you understand how "deductible" is defined in your policy. If you have a $250 deductible, for example, is that "per person," meaning that each family member has his or her own deductible to fulfill? Or, if your entire family is insured, do you get a break and only have to meet the deductible on perhaps two or three family members before coverage is provided for everyone? The latter option, of course, is the preferred one.

Remember to submit all your medical bills to your insurance company, even if you know that you haven't yet reached your deductible. Your insurer will keep track of these expenses, and as soon as they go over your deductible limit, your coverage will start.

The best rule of thumb is to take as large a deductible as you feel you can afford (especially if you are in excellent health and the likelihood of using your insurance to pay a claim is low).

SELECTING THE RIGHT CO-PAYMENT

Most fee-for-service policies establish a co-payment (or co-insurance) provision, often an 80–20 split, in which you pay 20 percent of your medical bills (over and above your deductible) while the insurer takes care of the remaining 80 percent. As with a deductible, your agreement to pay 20 percent of your medical costs is a way to help keep your premiums at a reasonable level.

However, when it comes to co-payments, you have another important decision to make: How much of a co-payment are you willing to assume? Avoid splits such as 90–10, which will keep your premiums very high. At the other end of the spectrum, if you can afford to pay perhaps 40 to 50 percent of your medical costs, you can dramatically reduce your premiums. Still, be cautious before agreeing to take on this much of a co-payment. If you become seriously ill, your medical costs can rise very high very quickly; if you're responsible for a 40 to 50 percent portion of, say, $20,000 in medical bills, that could be a devastating strain on your budget. The bottom line: For most people, an 80-20 split is probably the best compromise.

WILL "STOP LOSS" HELP?

Let's say you've finally found what you think is a good policy. It provides comprehensive benefits with manageable premiums, and calls for a $500 deductible and an 80–20 co-payment schedule. All is well—until you're involved in a bad automobile accident that puts you in the hospital for two weeks, during which time you undergo two operations. When you're finally back home recuperating, you submit the hospital bill—a whopping $65,000—to your insurance company. Not long thereafter, you get a notice from your insurer reminding you that under your 80–20 co-payment provision, you are responsible for 20 percent of the medical bills. You start to shake. Punching buttons on your calculator, you realize that in addition to your $500 deductible, you need to come up with $12,900! Suddenly, the 80–20 split has turned into a real burden, and you're left wondering where you went wrong.

However, there is a way to avoid a situation like this and the panic that goes with it. Talk to your insurance agent about including a "stop loss" provision in your coverage, which could become one of the most important parts of your policy. It places an upper limit or "cap" on the medical costs for which you're responsible in a given year. In short, it protects you against a financial bloodbath in the face of enormous medical bills. With a stop loss limit, once your out-of-pocket expenses (deductible + co-payment) have reached a set dollar amount, your insurance company pays 100 percent of the rest of your medical bills that year.

Let's look again at the scenario we described above. What if your policy had included a $3,000 stop loss clause? After your $500 deductible, you would have been responsible for paying 20 percent of the next $12,500 in medical fees. At that point, you would have paid out a total of $3,000—the stop loss limit in your policy—and your insurer then would have taken over completely, covering the remainder of your $62,000 in full. What a relief!

Don't put yourself in a position of being financially ravaged by just one serious illness or injury. Yes, a stop loss provision will raise your premium (the lower your cap, the higher the cost). But we feel it is money well spent.

WHAT'S THE BEST CEILING FOR YOU?

Don't forget this important point: The purpose of insurance is to protect you against a bankrupting illness, so make sure that your insurance priorities are in order. More than anything, be certain you have covered yourself against the large medical bills, even if it means paying the small ones yourself.

As part of that strategy, examine the "maximum coverage" provision of the policy that you're considering purchasing. In most cases, this is defined as the maximum amount of money that any one policy will pay over a lifetime. Once that level is reached, the insurance company will do a fast retreat, leaving you holding the remaining stack of medical bills.

> *More than anything, be certain you have covered yourself against the large medical bills, even if it means paying the small ones yourself.*

Simply because medical care is so costly, you need to make sure you're well protected by this provision. As a minimum, look for a cap of $1 million per person in lifetime benefits. If the policy provides for less—perhaps $250,000 or $500,000—you could be in trouble in the event of a catastrophic or chronic illness. And here's the good news: Raising your maximum benefit will not translate into a large increase in your monthly premium.

To repeat, make sure you're covered for the big bills. If you have a so-called "comprehensive" policy, it probably covers you not only for basic hospital-surgical costs, but also "major medical" (or catastrophic) insurance. The latter component generally has a large maximum benefit. In fact, if your personal budget won't allow you to spend too much on health insurance, look for a "major medical" policy before anything else. You might have to cover the first $500, $1,000, $2,000 or even $5,000 in medical costs yourself, but after that, you'll be protected up to $1 million or more. A good major medical policy will guard you against the costs of health catastrophes while not breaking your personal bank when you pay the premiums.

AVOID DUPLICATE COVERAGE

You already pay enough for your health insurance. Don't make the situation even worse by duplicating your coverage.

Let's say that both you and your spouse are employed and are provided group policies at work. You might think that with two policies, you're covered for everything—and more. But read the fine print. Most policies include a "limitation of benefits" clause that limits your reimbursement to 100 percent of the claim. In some cases, this clause actually disallows two companies from paying any part of the same claim. Thus, the value of a second policy, if any, is usually small; if you're paying premiums on two policies, you're probably wasting a lot of money.

So which policy do you choose—yours or your spouse's? You'll need to compare the benefits and premiums of each policy. Does one have a better co-payment provision than the other? Are the premiums considerably lower on one of them? Does one policy eliminate coverage for certain "pre-existing conditions," while the other does not?

Also, find out from the insurance administrators how much flexibility you have in choosing only partial coverage from one policy or the other. For instance, while you may decline the major medical coverage at your own job, ask if you can still subscribe to some other benefits—perhaps dental or vision care—that might not be part of your spouse's policy. Try to fill in any gaps that might exist this way.

Before you make the decision to turn down coverage at one workplace or the other, make sure you can participate in it at a later date. After all, if your spouse loses her job, and the family has been relying on her insurance plan, you need to be able to return to your own worksite's policy and reactivate it. While a laid-off worker has other options available (see a discussion of COBRA on page 31), the best alternative is usually to turn to another group plan.

One other thought on the subject of duplication: Avoid buying additional, separate policies—like accident insurance or cancer insurance—that are very specific in what they cover. If you have good health care coverage, you are probably already protected for any major disease, whether it's cancer, heart disease or arthritis. You'll just be throwing away your money by buying separate protection for cancer care, or for anything else, for that matter. The old cliche, "Some is good, more is better," doesn't necessarily apply when it comes to health insurance. Yes, you need coverage, but not just for cancer care or for treatment if you're injured falling on a slippery sidewalk. These disease-specific or accident policies are expensive and aren't worth much for most people.

HOW TO GET MORE INFORMATION

If the thought of comparing policies leaves you in a sweat, know that there's help available. One of the newest and easiest ways to compare insurance is via your computer. Several services have databases brimming with information on thousands of policies offered by hundreds of insurance companies. It's a simple way to see what policies offer in terms of price and benefits in a personalized format for you and your family.

A company called Quotesmith, for example, has information on coverage offered by any of 350 insurance companies that provide individual and group health insurance, Medicare supplemental insurance, long-term care insurance, and dental insurance. You'll receive a printout of what each policy includes and how much it costs, individualized to your age, family makeup, health status, and so on. You'll get pages of information that could help save you a lot of money. And, best of all, it's inexpensive. For $15, you can receive a market analysis of those policies that meet the criteria that you've provided. To contact Quotesmith, call 800-556-9393.

Quotesmith provides information for both individual and group insurance. Other database companies offer their services exclusively to corporations or insurance agents. One of them, Group Benefit Shoppers, won't do any price and benefit comparisons for you directly, but it will refer you to an insurance agent in your area who utilizes its software. You can contact Group Benefit Shoppers at 800-231-8495.

Getting the Most Out of Your Policy

Once you have made all your insurance decisions, written your first premium check, and received your policy in the mail (or from the insurance administrator at your work), your job isn't done yet. It's time to do some reading. You need to familiarize yourself with your entire policy, and make sure that the provisions you expected are really there.

Even after you purchase health insurance, most companies will give you a trial period to change your mind. This is particularly comforting if you bought your policy from a high-pressure insurance salesman who overwhelmed you with a blur of promises that you still don't fully understand. In some states, laws mandate a trial period of up to 30 days. During this time, if you're not satisfied with the policy, you can cancel your coverage and receive a full refund of your premium. Don't let this "free look" period lapse without deciding for sure whether you want to keep the insurance. Once the trial period is over, it's too late to cancel the policy without penalty.

Whether you have group or individual insurance, you may be notified periodically of changes in your coverage, particularly at renewal times. The administrator of the policy may provide you with a summary, either verbal or written, of the changes. However, ask to see more. Obtain a copy of the new policy itself and read it carefully. The more you know about your coverage, the better.

GETTING WHAT YOU PAY FOR

With HMOs, you probably won't have any health insurance forms to fill out and submit. That's one of their real advantages. By contrast, with fee-for-service plans, you need to take responsibility for getting all the necessary paperwork filled out and turned in. Otherwise, your doctor won't get paid or you won't get reimbursed. Every year, insurance companies save millions of dollars because of the "nuisance factor"—that is, claims are never paid because people thought it was too much trouble to file their claim forms.

Obviously, that's not a very practical way to utilize (or, more accurately, not utilize) your insurance. If you're going to pay for coverage, you might as well use it. Make sure you understand the time limits on filing claims.

Indemnity Policies: Worth the Price?

From time to time, you may receive solicitations in the mail, selling health insurance called "indemnity policies." These policies usually provide hospitalization coverage, but not in a traditional format. Instead, they offer a fixed payment for every day you are in the hospital—and usually the payment is so low that it covers only a small portion of your actual hospitalization costs.

For example, a hospital might charge you $700 a day for room, board and miscellaneous services. An indemnity policy, however, is more likely to pay you just $100, $200 or $300 a day while you're hospitalized. That will leave you with a shortfall of $400 a day or more that's not covered.

Unless you can't get any other kind of health insurance, these indemnity policies don't make sense. They are often overpriced for the benefits they provide. Spend your health insurance dollars somewhere else.

Every year, insurance companies save millions of dollars because of the "nuisance factor"—that is, claims are never paid because people thought it was too much trouble to file their claim forms.

Some policies require that you obtain your insurance company's permission before you have major medical procedures, from elective operations to, in some instances, even emergency hospital treatment. If you don't get permission ahead of time, your medical bills might not be covered. When you sign up for a policy, make sure you understand what is expected and the best way to abide by these guidelines.

If you ever find yourself in a situation where a claim is denied, go through the appeals process that your insurer should already have in place. Ask for a written explanation of why the claim was turned down. Point to the provisions in your policy that you believe cover the care you received. If you're convinced that you're right, don't give in. Write letters. Don't hesitate to enlist your doctor's support. If your claim was rejected on the presumption that it was not medically necessary, who better to come to your defense than the doctor who prescribed the test or treatment? Ask him or her to explain to the insurance company why the care was appropriate and important.

SWITCHING INSURANCE PLANS

If you ever decide to switch health insurance policies, perhaps because you've grown unhappy with the coverage or the service of your current insurer, do so cautiously. More than anything, don't drop your current policy and leave yourself uninsured while you're looking for other coverage. Keep in mind that new policies may have a waiting period before some of their benefits kick in. Before you discontinue one policy, make sure you can live with the provisions of the new one.

Sometimes, of course, the need to change insurance isn't your idea. If you are laid off, quit your job or retire, or if the business you work for closes down, you'll be faced with a lot of life changes, not the least of which is the need to decide how to keep your family's health protected.

If you have group insurance, things will change when you're no longer part of the group. Even so, you won't be left out in the cold, thanks to Congress' passage of the Consolidated Omnibus Budget Reconciliation Act (COBRA) of 1985, which helps protect people who lose their jobs, and applies to companies with 20 or more employees. Under the provisions of COBRA, you can get "continuation coverage" on your group health insurance (fee-for-service or managed care) for up to 18 months (or up to 36 months if you lose protection because of death, divorce or separation). However, you are responsible for paying the entire cost of the premiums for this insurance, plus a small fee (up to 2 percent of the premium) to cover the administrative costs incurred by your employer. You'll keep the same coverage, and the price of your premium will be no more than 102 percent of the price paid by your former co-workers.

What happens once the 18- (or 36-) month period passes? You can be dropped from the group policy at that time or have your premiums raised substantially. By then, however, you should have found either another job with group health insurance of its own, or an individual policy that is affordable and fits your needs.

In this era when job security is as obsolete as the Model T—and thus the chances of losing your group coverage are real—it's important to understand some other provisions of COBRA:

- If you were fired from your job because of "gross misconduct," your employer is not obligated to offer you continuation coverage.

- Once you leave your job, you have a 60-day "window" in which to decide whether or not to use COBRA. For example, let's say that you initially decline continuation coverage, only to change your mind two, four or six weeks later. As long as you let your old employer know of your decision within 60 days of your job loss, you have the right to reactivate your group coverage.

- To receive continuation coverage, you do not need to take a physical examination or go through any new waiting period before pre-existing conditions are covered.

- If you worked for a company with fewer than 20 employees, COBRA does not apply. However, some states have laws of their own, in which COBRA-like provisions protect people who lose their jobs.

Some Final Thoughts

With health insurance so costly, you still might be tempted to do without it, particularly if your family has always been pretty healthy. But that's a risk not worth taking. "Going bare" can ruin you financially if an unexpected and serious illness or injury occurs. Even so, according to recent studies, 32 million Americans have no health insurance at all, often because they simply can't afford it or because pre-existing illnesses have made them an unwelcome customer for any insurance company.

Even if it means cutting corners in other areas of your family budget, you need to set aside some money for health insurance. And buy it now rather than later. Many people put it off, figuring that they'll have more money next month or next year. If they're feeling well, they decide that doing without insurance is a simple way to reduce expenses. The problem is that you may not be feeling well tomorrow—and at that time, insurance may cost a lot more, or be impossible to get.

A Work Perk

As commonplace as work-based coverage is today, it wasn't always so accessible. In fact, employer-provided health insurance is a relatively new phenomenon, first taking root during World War II, when workers were offered medical coverage in lieu of pay raises. Overnight, health insurance became a valuable perk—a "plum" that still keeps many people hanging on to jobs they might have otherwise left years earlier.

HOW TO SAVE MONEY ON DOCTOR BILLS

Did you know that physicians' fees (charges for services the doctor provides directly to you) account for about 20 percent of the annual U.S. health care bill? This means, on average, about one out of every five dollars you spend for health care will end up in a doctor's hands, whether it's your personal physician or other consultants involved in your care. But that's not all. Physicians also control at least another 55 percent of all health care expenditures because they are the ones who admit patients to hospitals and nursing homes, prescribe medications, and order tests and procedures.

While none of these things can be done without your consent, you can't ignore the tremendous influence your doctor has on your health care decisions. In fact, next to keeping yourself healthy, finding the right doctor is the most important—and maybe the most difficult—step you can take in cutting your medical bills. For while the self-care and preventive measures you practice throughout your life can help reduce your use of the medical system, few people stay completely free of illness their entire lives. Our advice: You'd better have a trustworthy and cost-conscious doctor on your side if and when you do get sick. Your doctor will be the one who has the most influence on whether you start down the trail of testing and treatment or simply rest and sip chicken soup. Which direction you take could either save or cost you a fortune.

Why You Need a Primary Care Doctor

Today's health care system is extremely complicated, and it's easy to waste money if you don't know how to deal with it. If you really have serious medical problems, you could literally bankrupt yourself on the medical bills—even if you have insurance. Because your doctor plays a critical role in determining how efficiently you use the health care system, it's essential—before you get sick—to establish a good relationship with your primary care physician.

A primary care physician is interested in caring for the whole person, not a particular body system or medical specialty. Primary care physicians offer comprehensive medical care and advice on how to stay healthy, and serve as your advocate in all health-related matters. This includes explaining your options when it comes to tests and treatments, helping you find a specialist when you need one, coordinating all your care and keeping track of all your medications when more than one doctor is treating you at the same time. Probably the best way to assure that you receive high-quality health care at the best price is to find a primary care physician with whom you can develop a strong, ongoing relationship.

If you don't have a primary care doctor, you may be forced to meet your health care needs in a perpetual crisis mode. You get sick and there's no one to consult with by phone. You're not sure what kind of doctor to see, so you delay treatment and hope your problem goes away. When it doesn't, you get bounced from one specialist to another or, worse yet, you find yourself in a busy emergency room facing a harried physician who most likely wishes you weren't there. You end up with poor care at the highest possible price, simply because you didn't have a primary care physician who knew you and cared about you.

Where Do People See Doctors?

Generally, doctor-patient contacts are made in the following ways:

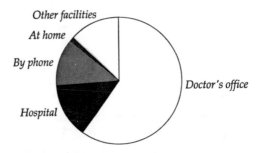

While a primary care physician generally doesn't have the specialized training needed to treat a cancer patient, prescribe glasses or remove a gallbladder, he or she does have the knowledge and ability to oversee your normal health maintenance and to know when referral to a specialist is necessary. If you do have a disease or condition requiring a specialist, the primary care doctor is the best person to coordinate your overall care, which includes keeping track of medications and tests and helping you communicate with the rest of the health care system.

> *Probably the best way to assure that you receive high-quality health care at the best price is to find a primary care physician with whom you can develop a strong, ongoing relationship.*

Even if you think of yourself as nontraditional and take an alternative approach to your health care, you still need to have a primary care physician you can call your own. Somewhere along the way, you're going to need traditional medicine in a hurry, and you'll do better for both your health and your pocketbook if you already have a primary care doctor you can turn to.

What Kind of Primary Care Provider Should You Choose?

Obviously, your primary care doctor should be a physician who is licensed to practice medicine by your state and is in "good standing" with your state's licensing board. (By good standing, we mean a doctor who is not on probation for violations of the law or for complaints related to incompetence.) To check on licenses and disciplinary problems, call your state medical licensing board.

TYPES OF PRIMARY CARE PROVIDERS

Primary care providers can be chosen from the following types of physicians:

FAMILY PHYSICIANS have completed medical school and a three-year residency in family practice. To become board-certified, they must pass a rigid exam administered by the American Board of Family Physicians. Then they must maintain their certification through regular continuing medical education activities.

Family physicians are trained to prevent, diagnose and treat a wide variety of ailments in patients of all ages. They have a broad range of training that includes surgery, psychiatry, internal medicine, obstetrics and gynecology, pediatrics and geriatrics. They place special emphasis on care of families on a continuing basis, using consultations and community resources when appropriate. They apply modern techniques to prevent, diagnose and treat the vast majority of common illnesses and injuries.

M.D. or D.O.—What's the Difference?

When selecting a primary care physician, one choice you'll have is between an M.D. (Doctor of Medicine) and a D.O. (Doctor of Osteopathy). Many years ago, the difference between the two could be very great, depending on where the doctors were trained. But in recent years, the education of both M.D.s and D.O.s has tended to be more similar than different. In fact, at some universities, the M.D. and D.O. candidates read the same textbooks and attend many of the same classes. At the internship and residency level, many D.O.s and M.D.s are working in the same programs.

There is, however, a basic philosophical difference in their training: D.O.s tend to emphasize a more holistic approach, although in practice they use the same diagnostic tests and therapies as M.D.s. The major difference is that a central part of the D.O. curriculum involves the use of the hands ("manipulation") in diagnosis and treatment.

Nationally, about five percent of all practicing physicians are graduates of osteopathy schools. The majority of D.O.s (approximately 60 percent) go into primary care, while only about 25 percent of M.D. graduates choose this type of practice. Whether you pick an M.D. or a D.O., it's important to find one whose training in primary care extends beyond medical school and internship and includes residency experience.

For more information about M.D.s, contact the American Medical Association at (312) 464-5000; for information about D.O.s, call the American Osteopathic Association at (800) 621-1773.

For more information on family physicians, contact the American Academy of Family Physicians at (816) 333-9700.

> *With time, most of the "old-time" general practitioners will likely be replaced by doctors who have trained in residency programs as family physicians.*

GENERAL PRACTITIONERS (GP's) offer the same care as family physicians, but have not completed a formal residency in family practice. Typically, GP's are older physicians whose years of experience may offset their lack of residency training. Before the specialty of family practice was "invented," many physicians became general practitioners. With time, most of the "old-time" general practitioners will likely be replaced by doctors who have trained in residency programs as family physicians.

Some older "GP's" have passed the examination of the American Board of Family Physicians and have been certified without having completed a formal residency program. If you are considering a general practitioner, we recommend that you choose a physician who is certified by the American Board of Family Practice.

INTERNISTS are physicians who have completed at least a three-year residency in general internal medicine. However, unlike family physicians, internists do not treat children or deliver babies. An internist is either a generalist (functioning as a primary care doctor for adults) or a specialist who completes additional training in a subject such as cardiology or pulmonary disease.

Internists must pass a certifying exam, administered by the American Board of Internal Medicine, and complete annual continuing education activities in order to maintain board certification.

An adult who has a chronic condition might want to use an internist as a primary care physician. For example, if you are seeing an internist because you have heart disease or arthritis, he or she might be the most appropriate doctor to go to for your primary care. Because this doctor is familiar with your chronic condition, he or she may offer the most efficient and cost-effective solution for all your care. However, many internists who subspecialize do not provide primary care, so you'll need to discuss this option with the doctor. Also, a subspecialist may be more expensive than your general internist, so you should talk about costs before using this type of physician for all your general medical needs.

For more information on internists, call the American College of Physicians at (215) 351-2400.

PEDIATRICIANS specialize in the care of children (but they do not perform surgery or deliver babies). If you choose a family physician as the primary provider for your family, that doctor will consult a pediatrician if your child becomes seriously ill or complex problems arise.

You may want to use a pediatrician from the start as your child's primary care physician. Before making your decision, you should compare the charges of the pediatricians and family physicians you are considering for the same type of services (for example, routine visits, immunizations, emergency visits). Pediatricians complete approved residency programs and are board-certified by the American Academy of Pediatrics through a qualifying exam and ongoing continuing education programs.

For more information, contact the American Academy of Pediatrics at (708) 228-5005.

OBSTETRICIANS/GYNECOLOGISTS (OB-GYNs) are trained in the medical and surgical care of the female reproductive system and associated disorders. They are also the doctors who most commonly deliver babies. Though not usually included in a list of primary care providers, they often serve as primary care physicians for women, and some are willing to treat minor medical problems that are not gynecologic in nature. If you wish to use your Ob-Gyn this way, you should discuss it thoroughly with the doctor to determine what conditions he or she is willing to treat and how much extra will be charged for this care.

While relying on your gynecologist as your primary provider of medical care might be acceptable if you are a generally healthy woman, you should realize that doctors in this specialty are not trained specifically to treat high blood pressure, diabetes and many other chronic conditions.

If you use a family physician or internist for primary care, a visit to an Ob-Gyn should be unnecessary unless you have specific problems that require a gynecological or obstetrical consultation. Your family physician or internist should be doing your pelvic examinations, Pap tests and breast exams.

An obstetrician/gynecologist completes an approved four-year residency program and passes a certifying exam of the American Board of Obstetrics and Gynecology. Board certification is a requirement for membership in the American College of Obstetricians and Gynecologists.

> *If you use a family physician or internist for primary care, a visit to an Ob-Gyn should be unnecessary unless you have specific problems that require a gynecological or obstetrical consultation.*

For additional information, contact the American College of Obstetricians and Gynecologists at (202) 638-5577.

WHEN TO USE A SPECIALIST

For serious and complex medical problems, specialists are usually better prepared to handle the diagnosis and treatment—at least initially. However, this is not true for most routine medical care or for the management of minor medical problems. Specialists usually charge more, tend to order expensive tests, and generally rely more on expensive and time-consuming procedures. For this reason, you should use your primary care physician except when a specific problem makes it necessary to see a specialist.

When your problem is more complex than your primary care provider can handle, he or she will help you select a specialist. An exception to this might be a visit to an optometrist or ophthalmologist for your routine eye exam. Even then, a phone call to your primary care provider may be the best first step in choosing a specialist.

Some people make the mistake of running from specialist to specialist for their medical needs. This approach not only costs more—it exposes you to unnecessary risk and decreases the quality of your care.

For example, let's say you develop a chronic headache. Who should you see for a diagnosis and treatment? A neurologist? An endocrinologist? A radiologist? A psychiatrist? Headaches can be caused by a variety of conditions, ranging from something as serious as a brain tumor to something as minor as the wrong eyeglass prescription.

Should you have an expensive brain scan? What should be done next? Making the right decision about which tests and treatments you receive can have a major impact on the final cost of your medical care and how quickly your suffering is relieved. Your primary care physician, who is familiar with your complete medical history, is in the best position to diagnose and treat minor problems. When that approach doesn't work, he or she is the best person to determine which specialist you should see for further testing and treatment.

Types of Practices

There are several types of practices in which doctors see patients, and each type has certain characteristics that can affect how satisfied you

How to Tell If Your Doctor Is Board-Certified

Once you determine the type of primary care provider that best fits your needs, you should then add another criterion: certification by a medical specialty board. After physicians have completed residency training, they are eligible to take the "board" exams for that specialty. Once they pass the exam, these doctors are entitled to call themselves "board-certified," which means they have proven their knowledge and skills in their chosen specialty. While not an absolute guarantee of competence, board certification is generally a good indicator of a physician's expertise. Physicians who have completed a residency but not taken or passed the exam yet are considered "board-eligible." If a doctor remains board-eligible for more than a year or two, you should consider the possibility that he or she has failed the board exam. This is the most common reason why a doctor would not go on to be board-certified within two or three years.

When checking a physician's board status, don't be swayed by the physician's listing in the yellow pages of the phone book. The specialty-by-specialty breakdown has no bearing on whether or not an individual is "board-certified" or has any specific training in that specialty area. Legally, a physician can choose to list under any specialty heading, regardless of training.

are with your care and what you'll end up paying. Before you choose a doctor, you also need to understand the different kinds of practices and how they affect patients.

SOLO PRACTICE OR GROUP PRACTICE?

A solo practitioner is a single physician who sets up his or her own office (like most doctors used to do in the "old days") and maintains a relationship with other physicians for patient coverage on weekends, nights and vacations. Today, more doctors choose to practice in groups, which may be made up of the same or different specialities. While each physician sees his or her own patients, group members cover off-hours for one another.

In fact, the yellow-page listing can be quite confusing and misleading.

To determine a prospective doctor's status, ask the physician or office staff about board certification. If you have any doubt, go to the public library and look up the doctor in The Directory of Medical Specialists. This book will give updated information on board certification of all specialties and is an excellent resource.

To check a doctor's board status by phone, use the following numbers:

American Board of Medical Specialties: 1-800-776-CERT (This toll-free hotline enables you to check certification of physicians in any specialty.)

You can also call the specialty board listings below to determine a doctor's certification status:

American Board of Family Practice: (606) 269-5626

American Board of Internal Medicine: (215) 243-1500

American Board of Pediatrics: (919) 929-0461

American Board of Obstetrics and Gynecology: (214) 871-1619.

> *"Fee-for-service" doctors itemize their bills and charge for each service they provide according to a set schedule of fees.*

Remembering the importance of your relationship with your primary care physician, you should consider how a doctor's type of practice might influence that relationship. If your doctor practices in a group or is part of an HMO, how likely are you to see that doctor at each visit? How often is your doctor gone, whether it's for vacation or for medical meetings? Who covers when he or she is gone? How many different doctors rotate coverage? Does the covering doctor have access to your records? Before you choose a doctor as your own, you should know the answers to all of these questions.

HOW WILL YOU PAY?

There are a number of ways in which doctors are paid. While we go into more detail on the types of plans in Chapter 1, here's a review of the most common payment structures.

FEE-FOR-SERVICE—In this approach, doctors itemize their bills and charge for each service they provide according to a set schedule of fees. These could be paid by you, by your insurance plan, or by both of you combined. If you have an "indemnity" type of insurance policy, you're free to consult any "fee-for-service" doctor, although you will probably be responsible for paying a portion of the doctor's charges.

PPO (PREFERRED PROVIDER ORGANIZATION)—Doctors who are members of preferred provider organizations have agreed to provide services according to a fee schedule established by a participating insurer. In PPO plans, your insurer will usually pay all or most of your physician expenses as long as you use participating physicians. In some cases, you will be required to make a co-payment, usually a small percentage of the total bill. PPO plans offer a list of participating doctors to choose from, so you have some degree of freedom in the choice of a physician. However, if you're already happy seeing a non-participating physician, this plan will penalize you financially for using that doctor's services. The only way around this problem is to convince your doctor to become a participant in the plan and to accept the plan's payment schedule.

HMO (HEALTH MAINTENANCE ORGANIZATION)—HMO plans are the fastest-growing method of providing health care in the United States. In an HMO, all of the medical needs of members are met for a prede- termined (usually prepaid) monthly or annual fee. Sometimes the fee is paid by the employer, sometimes by individuals, and sometimes it is shared.

HMOs can be organized "under one roof," where all of the physi- cians are employees of the HMO, or through "individual practice associations" (IPAs), where the HMO contracts with private physi- cians or groups of doctors to take care of insured subscribers.

While HMO patients are offered some choice of physicians, it is usu- ally limited to those doctors who are approved by the HMO. These doctors agree to follow certain guidelines established by the HMO, including some that could restrict your access to certain tests, drugs or procedures within the HMO.

HMOs often utilize nurse practitioners and physician assistants to perform functions that are usually done by physicians, such as Pap exams and prenatal visits. These individuals have more training than a registered nurse, but considerably less than a doctor, so they always work under a doctor's supervision. This frees doctors for more com- plicated and serious cases. Nurse practitioners, for example, are often used in obstetrics and gynecology for routine prenatal care and rou- tine pelvic examinations. In the pediatric area, they may take care of well-baby visits and exams. Some private practices also use these indi- viduals, not only to hold down physician costs but because patients like them—they take more time than doctors to listen and to teach.

Should you choose an HMO, you'll be less concerned with cost (since your monthly payment should cover all or almost all of your costs, regardless of how often you use the services) and more concerned with getting all the care you need. In some HMOs, physicians are evaluated and rewarded for increasing their "efficiency" and saving the HMO money. Sometimes, that translates into keeping you from getting the service you need. This, of course, is the opposite of fee-for-service practice, where a physician makes more money by doing more for or to you.

CLINICS—Today, clinics come in all shapes and sizes. The most impor- tant thing to understand about clinics is that the word "clinic" does

> *The most important thing to understand about clinics is that the word "clinic" does not automatically mean a public or low-cost facility.*

not automatically mean a public or low-cost facility. In fact, clinics vary tremendously in the quality and type of care they provide.

PRIVATE CLINICS—Private clinics are pretty much the same as group practices; however, they usually have more than one specialty and some testing facilities on the clinic premises. Also, private clinics often have special relationships with area hospitals. Most clinics listed in the phone book (especially in the yellow pages) are private and offer no financial advantages to you. Some private clinics operate as mini-HMOs, providing patients with outpatient services for a set monthly fee. If you decide to use a clinic, be sure you determine in advance exactly how you will be charged for all of the services rendered and to what extent your insurance will cover those charges.

Some privately funded clinics that were created to serve low-income patients frequently offer services to others on a sliding scale. Typically, these clinics were established to provide a specific kind of care (for example, prenatal or well-baby care). One example of a privately funded clinic is Planned Parenthood, which offers high-quality gynecological care and counseling to all women, and is an excellent resource for any woman who cannot afford to see a private physician.

The best way to find out about these clinics is to call your county public health department or your state or county medical society.

PUBLIC CLINICS—Funded fully or partially by taxes, public clinics are often affiliated with large public hospitals or medical schools and can offer very good care, although you may encounter long waits to get that care, as well as bureaucratic paperwork and little choice of doctor. Services and fees vary widely in these clinics. Services are frequently offered on a sliding fee scale based on income level, which results in charges that are usually much less expensive than private care. Public clinics frequently include services for prenatal care and early childhood care (including vaccinations) free or at a very nominal charge. Additionally, public clinics periodically offer special screening services at no cost, including blood pressure measurements, pelvic examinations and Pap exams, as well as screening for high blood cholesterol and tuberculosis. Note that public clinics are not necessarily just for the poor. You should consider a public clinic if you are employed but uninsured or underinsured, or if you have a pre-existing medical condition that is not covered by your insurance. To find out about public clinics in your area, contact your state or county department of public health.

LOCAL MEDICAL AND DENTAL SCHOOLS—Another inexpensive or free way to obtain medical attention is by contacting local teaching facilities. These institutions often sponsor clinics where patients are treated by student residents and interns who are closely supervised by accredited physicians and dentists. Most schools now charge for their services, but the fees are often based on your ability to pay and may be substantially lower than treatment at private facilities.

How to Find the Right Doctor

Once you've determined the type of doctor and setting that best meet your needs, you need to figure out how to find the right doctor. Here are a few sources you can use for help and advice:

ASK FRIENDS AND FAMILY FOR RECOMMENDATIONS

Be very specific in the questions you ask. For example: Why do they like their doctor? What do they dislike? How much does the doctor charge? Do they think the doctor orders too many tests? Too few? Can they talk to the doctor comfortably about costs?

ASK OTHER HEALTH PROFESSIONALS FOR SUGGESTIONS

Nurses, lab technicians and medical secretaries get to see how doctors perform under many different circumstances. They have a good eye for a good doctor . . . as well as for a bad one.

ASK THE PERSON IN CHARGE OF HEALTH BENEFITS AT YOUR COMPANY OR CALL YOUR INSURANCE PROVIDER

They may offer a list of practitioners who have a reputation for delivering good care at a reasonable cost. Once you have some suggestions, check to see if any disciplinary action has been taken against the physician by contacting your state board of medical examiners. You can investigate malpractice claims that have not been settled or that are ongoing against the physician by contacting the county clerk's office where the doctor practices.

MAKE A PHONE CALL TO THE DOCTOR'S OFFICE

When you've narrowed down your list of candidates to two or three, conduct phone interviews with the office staff. Here are some key questions to include in your interview:

- Is the doctor taking new patients?
- Where did the doctor train and is he or she board-certified?
- At what hospital(s) does the doctor have privileges?
- How long does it take to get an appointment?
- Is the doctor punctual? What's the usual wait?
- Does the doctor qualify as a provider for your health plan?
- Will the office staff complete all insurance forms? Do they accept Medicare insurance assignment?
- What does the doctor charge for a complete physical and for an intermediate visit?
- What does the doctor do when a patient cannot afford to pay a bill? Ask if the office offers credit arrangements for payment.
- Does the doctor personally handle patient telephone calls of a medical nature?
- How does the doctor handle patient emergencies?
- Who covers for the doctor during off-hours (weekend, vacations, etc.)? How often is the doctor unavailable because of vacations, medical meetings or other commitments?

If your questions are answered clearly and concisely, ask if you can come in for a brief meeting with the doctor. This is the best way to determine if you are going to be comfortable with the doctor's communication style and general manner. Ask beforehand if there is a charge for this initial visit.

This interview should give you an indication of the doctor's interest in you and your opinions. Further, it offers you an opportunity to evalu-

ate the physician as an advisor and tea-
cher. Is he or she willing to spend the
time or do you feel rushed? Are questions answered in an understandable
fashion? Are your concerns treated with
respect? If you find that all accredita-
tions are in order, the interest and the
manner that the physician exhibits in
the interview should play a major role in
your decision.

> *Even the same doctor may charge different prices for different patients, depending on the patient's ability to pay or the kind of insurance coverage a patient has.*

Remember, you are a prospective client to a physician. And, physicians are often willing to deal with each patient, case-by-case, when it comes to care and fees. So, talk to the doctor about your medical needs and your financial needs. Most doctors will listen and many will work with you.

Don't hesitate to discuss money as part of your get-acquainted visit. It is appropriate and in your interest to make a financial arrangement in advance that works.

What Should a Doctor Charge

The prices that different doctors charge for the same procedure vary widely. Even the same doctor may charge different prices for different patients, depending on the patient's ability to pay or the kind of insurance coverage a patient has.

Just to remind you again: Higher prices do not necessarily mean better quality. In fact, some of the worst doctors in practice deliberately charge more than anyone else in their community to create the illusion that they are better. Anyone who falls for this trick gets cheated twice—on both cost and quality.

The differences between the lowest and the highest prices are impossible to explain on medical grounds. How can some pediatricians justify charging $60 for a DTP shot when the average cost is $35? (Answer: They can't.) How can some obstetricians justify a $5,500 bill for delivering a baby when the average doctor charges $2,000 and some doctors are willing to do it for $1,000? (Answer: They can't.) How can some ophthalmologists keep a straight face while charging $2,800

> If patients refused to pay excessive fees, the doctors would either lower their prices or retire.

more than their colleagues for a 20-minute cataract operation? (Answer: They must have no conscience.) And what kind of cardiac surgeon would charge $7,000 more than average for a coronary artery bypass operation? (Answer: A very greedy one.)

These doctors couldn't get away with these gross overcharges if their patients didn't let them. If patients refused to pay excessive fees, the doctors would either lower their prices or retire (we're guessing that most would lower their prices).

So why *do* patients keep coming and paying excessive fees? Many are simply unaware they can buy the same service for much less elsewhere. Some do so because their insurance covers the cost, so they don't care what the doctor charges (some day these folks will wake up and realize that they are paying for the high fees in the long run through higher insurance premiums). And still others believe that higher doctor charges mean better medical care. We'd like to correct that myth right now.

Our advice is simple: Before you see any physician for routine care or special procedures, make sure that the doctor's charges are fair and consistent with the customary charges in your community. Is the doctor on a "preferred provider" list approved by your insurance company? If not, you may personally have to pay not only the difference but also a larger percentage of the entire bill. If you choose to do so, be aware that there is no assurance you'll be getting any better care for the extra money.

ONCE YOU FIND A DOCTOR, PRACTICE RESTRAINT

Once you've chosen a physician, you're ready to practice ways to save money. The first—and best—way is by going to the doctor only when necessary. Some experts estimate that as many as 70 percent of all doctor visits for new problems are unnecessary since they are for minor ailments where patients would have gotten better anyway on their own. That's a lot of time and money spent on care that probably could have been given at home—at no charge.

The best way to keep yourself out of the doctor's office is to know as much as possible about your health. First, you should have a good medical guide book that helps you determine when a visit to the doctor is necessary. If you have an ongoing condition, read up on it and know what kind of medical care you need to best manage your condition.

Some experts estimate that as many as 70 percent of all doctor visits for new problems are unnecessary.

Two very helpful guides are *Take Care of Yourself* and *The American Medical Association's Family Medical Guide*. These books give you the information you need to make sound decisions on when to see a doctor. They include full descriptions of when checkups and standard tests are necessary.

All too often, people use the doctor's office for reassurance instead of medical care. That's understandable, but visiting the doctor when you're not really sick is an expensive way to get reassurance. Why not call first? If your doctor thinks your symptoms warrant an office visit, then it makes sense to go.

Basic Tips for Saving on Doctor Bills

Cost issues are not covered by medical school curricula, so physicians are generally not well versed on just how much the various components of health care cost. Quite frankly, cost is usually not a major factor in a physician's thinking. So, it's up to you. After all, you are the one paying the bill.

Tests, specialists, second opinions, medications—you need to know why and how much. You must make it very clear to your doctor that all of your health care is approached with finances in mind. You can't control your costs if you and your physician don't have this kind of relationship.

Only about one-third of all patients ever discuss money with their physicians. Some patients hesitate to discuss costs or to question tests, medications or other recommendations because they feel the doctor may be offended by their questions. This completely discounts the important role you play in your health care. However, it doesn't mean that you need to approach your doctor in an adversarial way. Quite the contrary, your doctor should realize that you are a very astute patient.

NEGOTIATE COSTS FOR ALL DOCTOR VISITS

Doctors frequently have different, unpublished fees for different patients. If the doctor is aware of your circumstances, he or she will

Where Does Your Doctor Fit In?

To give you an idea of what are reasonable and customary fees for physician office visits, look at the following information based on a survey by the American Medical Association. This chart shows fees for an established patient.

The Mean Fee (In Dollars) For a Physician Office Visit With an Established Patient

Area	All Physicians	GP/FP*	Internal Medicine	Surgery	Peds*	OB/GYN
National	42.08	33.35	43.72	42.74	40.02	49.07
New England	48.83	—	46.29	48.69	—	—
Mid-Atlantic	49.97	36.13	48.12	52.91	48.22	61.63
East North Central	36.53	29.96	38.35	35.19	34.56	44.54
West North Central	34.94	27.54	40.48	36.27	—	40.40
South Atlantic	41.45	33.90	41.60	41.94	39.31	46.98
East South Central	36.04	29.41	39.19	36.28	—	—
West South Central	36.31	30.97	40.54	34.00	33.77	42.01
Mountain	39.59	33.64	—	40.69	—	—
Pacific	47.51	39.50	49.54	48.86	43.44	53.55

*GP/FP = General Practitioner/Family Physician; *Peds = Pediatrician

Source: 1991 AMA Socioeconomic Monitoring System core survey. Copyright 1992, American Medical Association.

probably be willing to work with you on charges. Remember, your doctor's office is a place of business—where you are the client. Most doctors will not want to lose you as a patient; they'd rather work with you to come up with prices you can afford.

ASK ABOUT CASH DISCOUNTS

Many physicians offer cash discounts to people who pay their bills at the time the service is rendered—but you usually have to ask to get the discount.

WOULD THE DOCTOR WAIVE THE CO-PAYMENT?

If the co-payment portion of your insurance or Medicare presents a financial hardship to you or your family, discuss this with your doctor. He or she may be willing to waive that portion of the fee if you are unable to pay it after you have received the bill.

USE THE TELEPHONE

This is a great way to determine whether or not you need to go in for a visit. Be sure your doctor is willing to talk with you on the phone and offer good phone advice. In one study of middle-aged men with chronic conditions, phone advice made it possible for them to reduce their number of office visits by 19 percent; the overall cost of their medical care was reduced 28 percent.

STAY OUT OF THE EMERGENCY ROOM

In the ER, your bill will reflect the astronomical cost of maintaining a full-service department on a 24-hour basis. So, even if you go in for a runny nose, you're going to be paying a huge flat fee—just for walking in the door.

Except in real emergencies, stay away from emergency rooms. In most instances, your doctor should be able to help you if you need advice on an injury, and, if not available, should have another practitioner filling in. As a backup to your own doctor, investigate a free-standing medical facility, with extended hours, that can meet your needs in a nonhospital setting. These types of facilities can usually handle "minor emergencies"—simple stitches, setting a break, and so on—for a fraction of the cost of going to an emergency room. These facilities will be listed in the yellow pages of your phone book.

FOLLOW RECOMMENDATIONS FOR ANNUAL VISITS AND PREVENTIVE SCREENING TESTS

In many cases, screening recommendations have changed in recent years. Discuss the appropriate schedule of screening tests and exams with your physician or read about the subject in Chapter 9. For additional information you might want to consult *Take Care of Yourself* by Donald M. Vickery, M.D., and James F. Fries, M.D., or *The AMA's Family Medical Guide*.

BE SURE YOUR DOCTOR ORDERS TESTS FOR THE RIGHT REASONS

Are your tests being ordered to help make your diagnosis or to help your therapy—or as protection against malpractice claims? The best way to protect yourself from unnecessary tests or procedures is to ask questions. For more information on how to find out if you're getting the right test for the right reason, see Chapter 3.

GET A SECOND OPINION

Surgery or other procedures can be very expensive, not to mention risky, so agree to them only when you're absolutely sure they're needed. If your doctor suggests surgery or any other invasive procedure, get a second opinion prior to consenting.

A Cornell study found that second opinions for elective surgery saved up to $2.63 for every dollar spent on getting the second opinion. The procedures where the greatest cost savings were realized were hysterectomy, prostatectomy, bunionectomy, knee surgery, breast mass excision, deviated septum, hernia repair, cataract surgery and D&C (dilatation & curettage). For other procedures, such as coronary artery bypass and cholecystectomy, there were not enough patients in the study for the researchers to come to any conclusion.

How do you find a doctor to give you a second opinion? Check with your insurance company. Ask if second opinions are covered;

some insurance companies require second opinions for expensive procedures, and will have lists of doctors they can refer you to. As an alternative for people on Medicare, the Health Care Financing Administration operates a second-opinion hotline. Medicare recipients can call 1-800-638-6833 for help in finding a physician for a second opinion.

What should you do if the second doctor gives you an opinion that differs from the first? The two doctors should talk to each other to resolve the issue. Another option is to get yet a third opinion from another doctor. This may be necessary in any case if there is an insurance company deciding whether or not to pay for your surgery.

WHAT TO DO WHEN YOU VISIT THE DOCTOR

• When you go to the doctor, get the most you can out of the visit. If you have got a medical problem, take time before the visit to write out a brief history of what's been happening. What's the main problem as you see it? When did it begin? How has it affected you? What other problems relate to it? How have you handled it? Have you taken anything (medications) for it? Have you had any similar episodes in the past?

• Take notes while talking with the doctor. Ask the doctor to write down specific instructions, when necessary. Discuss any recommended tests, procedures or treatments and ask for the specific reason for the test—and the cost. Remember, you're buying this service and need to know what it's going to cost you. Question the doctor about any less expensive options. Make sure the doctor understands that you want to approve all tests prior to having them done. When prescriptions are necessary, be sure you and the doctor discuss the cost and alternatives (See Chapter 4).

• Always request an itemized bill. One of the main areas for mistakes in physician billing appear in the codes used in the itemization. A detailed bill will help you spot any errors and let you know exactly what you're paying for.

• Finally, if the doctor is not meeting your needs, find a new doctor. If every visit results in tests or prescriptions, re-evaluate your doctor. If you wait more than 15 minutes for appointments, complain to the doctor. If your doctor approaches your visits "on the run," find another doctor. If the actual bill is far more than the estimated costs, protest the charges. Remember, you are in charge and there are many other doctors out there interested in your valuable business.

When you leave your doctor's office, whether it was for a routine checkup or for a specific complaint, you should feel that you've spent time with a trusted professional and that you've had the opportunity to discuss what's on your mind. You should feel that the doctor answered your questions, explained all procedures or medications, and discussed prevention in a way that was understandable and specific to your situation. Most of all, you should feel that the money you spent was well spent and that you got what you needed from your visit.

HOW TO SAVE MONEY ON MEDICAL TESTS

How many blood tests, x-rays or other tests have you had lately? Doctors are ordering more tests than ever before. While there are some legitimate explanations for this, there are also some not so legitimate reasons. As you'll soon see, your doctor may be ordering tests for reasons that have very little to do with your illness or its treatment. One way or another, the cost of these questionable tests may be coming out of your pocket, as well as creating a potential threat to your health. In this chapter, we'll show you how you can avoid unnecessary tests and save money on the tests you do need.

"Why Would a Doctor Order Tests You Don't Need?"

Don't assume that just because your doctor orders a test, it's absolutely necessary. You may be surprised at some of the underlying reasons a test may be ordered—reasons that have little to do with "good medicine." Here are a few.

"DEFENSIVE" MEDICINE

Many doctors believe that the best way to defend themselves against a lawsuit is to order every test they can think of, even if that means ordering some tests that are not likely to yield useful results.

If that sounds unreasonable, put yourself in the doctor's shoes: Imagine yourself on a witness stand, being questioned by a hostile attorney about a certain medical test you had failed to order. You have to justify why you neglected to use every available tool, while the jury is likely to be sympathetic with the patient.

In reality, a doctor is probably much less likely to get sued by ordering only the tests necessary and keeping the patient fully informed about what's going on. This is simply good medical practice. Unfortunately, in today's legal environment, that doesn't sound like enough protection to many physicians.

Defensive medicine not only increases your costs, but the unnecessary tests could expose you to additional risks. This happens because the tests themselves may cause side effects or complications—like an allergic reaction when dye is injected into the bloodstream for a kidney x-ray or excessive bleeding after a biopsy is taken. In some cases, the risk from a test occurs because of a "false positive" result (this term is used to describe an inaccurate test result that says you've got a problem when you don't). Because of the erroneous report, you could end up having more tests with even greater risks. For example:

> Your doctor orders a "PSA" blood test to screen for prostate cancer (which you don't have). The lab makes an error and reports your PSA level as abnormally high, suggesting that a cancer is growing in your prostate gland. Your doctor then recommends that biopsies be taken from your prostate gland. The biopsies show no cancer, but you develop an infection at a biopsy site.

Though no one ever wants to go through an experience like the one described above, it's a lot easier to justify if the PSA test was really necessary. That would be the case if you were over 50 years old and the doctor discovered an enlarged area on your prostate gland, but it's a different matter if you're a relatively young man with a normal prostate gland and the doctor is simply practicing defensive medicine.

"SHORT-CUT" MEDICINE

Some doctors substitute a long list of laboratory tests and x-rays for a thorough history and physical, hoping that the tests will reveal a diagnosis that incomplete questioning and examination missed.

The overwhelming majority of medical problems, perhaps as many as 90 percent, can be diagnosed with a medical history and physical examination, followed by one or two carefully selected laboratory tests. But it takes a lot of time to do a complete history, which includes a discussion of your symptoms and all possible causes for them. And it takes a lot of time to do a complete physical examination—more time than some doctors are willing or able to spend.

"PASSIVE" MEDICINE

With increasing frequency, doctors are ordering tests just because patients ask for them. Sometimes, the patient's request makes sense: for example, when a woman over 50 asks for a screening mammogram or a man with high blood cholesterol asks the doctor to see how much of the elevation is due to the so-called "bad cholesterol" (LDL cholesterol) and how much is due to the "good" HDL. But some requests are not medically justified, as when a woman who's had a normal pelvic exam asks for an ultrasound examination because she's afraid of ovarian cancer, or a young man in good health asks for a new prostate cancer screening test he just heard about.

"A Very Expensive Pair of New Glasses"

A good example of "short-cut" medicine involved a member of our family, whose doctor advised her to have an MRI (magnetic resonance imaging) scan of her brain to see if a tumor was present. She had been suffering from severe headaches that started suddenly about six weeks earlier, and were occurring every day, almost all day. The doctor asked her very few questions about the headaches and performed only a very brief physical exam before ordering the MRI test (which cost $1050).

We learned about her headaches just a day before she was to have the test, and asked her several questions, one of which was "Did you get new glasses just before the headaches started?" Her answer: "Yes." When asked if the glasses had bifocal lenses, her reply again was "Yes." Her responses to our questions led us to believe that the headaches were caused by her tendency to hold her head back stiffly all day as she peered through the bottom of the bifocals to read her mail and work at her computer. In spite of our suggestions, her doctor insisted that she have the brain scan. The scan was normal, and the headaches disappeared with neck-stretching exercises and some instructions on how to use bifocals. The moral of the story? Expensive tests are not always the best way to make a diagnosis.

> *Some doctors substitute a long list of laboratory tests and x-rays for a thorough history and physical.*

Why are people so eager to be tested? Usually, it's because of something they've read in the newspaper, seen on television or heard on the radio. All too often, these media reports exaggerate the benefits of the tests and fail to disclose all of the risks. To some extent, we physicians are also responsible for our patients' requests. We've raised hopes that almost anything can be diagnosed and cured today, and we've misled people into believing that modern tests are completely accurate and safe.

Remember, there is nothing wrong with asking or even demanding that a test be done when it is really appropriate for you. In this situation, your doctor should be willing to order it. However, when the test is inappropriate, your doctor should refuse your request and explain why. A good physician will do just that, but some doctors are not willing to argue with a patient over a test. They don't have or won't spend time to explain why the test shouldn't be done, so they give in and order the test.

What does that mean to you as a patient? The trouble with this type of "passive" medicine is that you not only get tests you don't need and risks that are unnecessary and bills you can't afford, but you also get a doctor who isn't honest with you. It may seem relatively unimportant when the issue is a simple lab test, but this dishonest style of communication could cause major difficulty for you when your medical problems are more serious and the stakes are higher.

"ACADEMIC" MEDICINE

Medical tests are sometimes ordered out of "academic interest"—especially if you have an unusual disorder. This occurs most commonly in medical schools and teaching hospitals, but it can happen in private practice, too. For example, your doctor may want to present your case to others or write about it some day.

When your medical problem is unusual or particularly interesting, it may be reasonable for the doctor to order tests that are not—strictly speaking—needed to manage your case, if it will help others to learn. However, such tests should never be ordered without your permission (you have an absolute right to refuse), and your doctor is obligated to tell you about any costs and risks associated with the tests.

If you do give permission to perform a test for academic reasons, you should not be charged for it. When the test is ordered for the benefit of others, someone else should pay for it, such as the hospital or the research grant that is funding your doctor's studies.

"HABITUAL" MEDICINE

For some doctors, excessive test ordering is simply the extension of a bad habit they developed during medical school, internship and residency. These were the medical students who ordered unnecessary tests to avoid embarrassment the next day if they forgot to order one that was important. They became the doctors who—20 years later—are still ordering unnecessary tests.

Some doctors simply haven't kept up with the changing times and changing medical policies. In 1950, most interns were required—as a matter of policy—to order chest x-rays on every patient who entered the hospital. Later, when research studies proved that this policy was generally wrong, hospitals stopped requiring routine chest x-rays. But old habits die hard, so some physicians are still ordering those x-rays 40 years later, even though there is no justification for it.

The same problem exists for some screening tests. Annual Pap tests were once recommended for all women, until studies showed that, in most cases, this was a waste of money. Yet some doctors are still performing Pap tests every year on every patient, running up the laboratory costs for these women and even adding extra charges to their own bills for "handling" the unnecessary tests.

When used properly, screening tests like Pap tests are extremely important because they can provide warnings about the development of serious medical problems like cervical cancer. Early detection allows your doctor to start treatment before the disease has progressed to a dangerous stage, which increases your chance of cure and decreases the overall cost of your treatment. Screening tests like blood cholesterol measurements have yet another benefit: They alert you to problems you may be able to reverse or prevent completely with appropriate action.

Why Do Physicians Order Laboratory Tests?*

Over a five-year period, Dr. George D. Lundberg, editor of *JAMA: Journal of the American Medical Association,* asked physicians and laboratory workers this question. Answers included the following:

Confirmation of clinical opinion
Diagnosis
Monitoring
Screening
Prognosis
Unavailability of previous test results
Previous abnormal result
Question of accuracy of previous test result
Patient/family pressure
Peer pressure
Pressure from recent articles
Personal reassurance
Patient/family reassurance
Public relations
Ease of performance with ready availability
Hospital policy
Legal requirement
Documentation
Personal profit
Hospital profit
Attempt to defraud
Research
Curiosity
Insecurity
Frustration at nothing else to do
To buy time
Hunting or fishing expedition
To establish a baseline
To complete a data base
Personal education
To report to an attending physician
Habit

As you can see from this list, doctors do not always order tests with the best interests of your health or your wallet in mind.

*Source: JAMA: Journal of the American Medical Association, *February 4, 1983,* Volume 249, page 639. Copyright 1983, American Medical Association.

But there is a point of diminishing returns with most screening procedures, so getting tested too often will only increase your medical bills without significantly improving your chance of early diagnosis. In Chapter 9, you will find guidelines for how often the most commonly recommended screening tests should be done. These guidelines were developed by the federal government, by national health organizations like the American Cancer Society and American Heart Association, and by medical professional groups like the American Academy of Pediatrics and the American College of Obstetricians and Gynecologists. If your physician's recommendations for screening tests differ from these guidelines, you should ask the doctor why.

"MONETARY" MEDICINE

Did you know that your physician may have a financial interest in ordering more or fewer tests than you need?

For example, doctors who own laboratories or diagnostic imaging facilities (with x-ray or MRI machines) make more money by ordering more tests, while some doctors who work in prepaid insurance plans or HMOs may make more money by ordering fewer tests.

Doctors are professionals and they are supposed to resist potential conflicts of interest by using objective scientific criteria to decide when medical tests should be ordered. But doctors are only human, which means that some of them—not many, but some—will order unnecessary tests because they make more money doing so. And some doctors—not many, but some—may fail to order tests that should be done because their medical group is "over budget" and the year-end deficit will come out of their own pockets.

Because of the opportunity for abuse when physicians have a financial interest in a testing facility, federal regulations prohibit doctors from referring Medicare patients to any such facility (since the government is paying the bill, it gets to set the rules for these patients). To protect against abuse in non-Medicare patients, several states have passed regulations requiring physicians to disclose any financial interest they have in facilities to which they refer patients. Typically, doctors are required to notify you in writing that they have such an interest.

There are several important exceptions to these regulations—the most obvious being the laboratories, x-ray machines and other testing devices that practicing physicians operate in their own offices. It is neither illegal nor unethical for doctors to process patients' blood and urine specimens in their own office laboratories, and they are perfectly free to charge whatever they please for the tests they perform on these specimens. And there is no law or ethical restriction that prevents physicians from ordering x-rays or ultrasound tests, then doing these tests themselves, again charging whatever the traffic will bear. In fact, laboratories, x-ray machines and other diagnostic devices are a significant source of profit in many doctors' offices and clinics.

Doctors who run their own laboratories and perform their own x-ray and ultrasound procedures defend these practices on several grounds. They say that the labs and test facilities in their offices are a tremendous convenience to patients. Some say that lab tests and diagnostic procedures done in their offices are less expensive than those done by outside laboratories and specialists. This may be true in some cases, but there is no evidence that this is universally true, and—in fact—procedures done in doctors' offices are actually often more expensive than those done outside.

Perhaps the most important issue you need to be concerned about is the *quality* of the testing process and the accuracy of the results.

X-rays for Profit

A study reported in *The New England Journal of Medicine* in December, 1990, suggested that financial issues may have a significant impact on the use of selected tests by some physicians. Researchers compared the number of x-ray tests ordered by two different groups of practicing physicians: One group had their own x-ray machines in their offices and the other group sent all of their patients to outside radiologists for x-rays. The doctors who took their own x-rays (and kept the money charged for these x-rays) ordered more than four times as many x-ray tests as the doctors who sent their patients to the outside specialists.

Doctors' office laboratories are generally not held to the same strict standards as larger laboratories that are licensed to do work for others. The larger laboratories are tested and inspected at regular intervals by state authorities, while most labs in doctors' offices are not subjected to the same kind of scrutiny. Furthermore, except in the largest clinics and medical group labs, the personnel hired generally do not have the same advanced training and certification as the people in outside professional laboratories and diagnostic facilities.

> *Doctors' office laboratories are generally not held to the same strict standards as larger laboratories that are licensed to do work for others.*

Some tests can—and should—be done in the doctor's office, such as urinalysis, hematocrit (a quick measure of red blood cells) and examination of specimens under the microscope for bacteria and fungi. There are many other tests that can be done as accurately in most doctors' offices as in the laboratory—if the proper equipment is available, the technicians are properly trained and the doctor is capable of interpreting the results. These tests include blood sugar and blood cholesterol measurements and some x-rays or ultrasound tests.

But some tests are best not done in the average doctor's office. For example, mammograms should only be done in facilities that are certified by the American College of Radiology. The facility should have a dedicated machine (this means that the x-ray apparatus is specifically set for performing mammograms and not used for anything else). And mammograms should be "read" (interpreted) only by radiologists who are specially trained for this task. If you settle for anything else, you risk the possibility that a very early cancer will be missed.

NEW TECHNOLOGY

A common cause of excessive testing is that new tests are constantly being developed. While new technology can be exciting, the equipment can be quite costly and this cost is passed on to the patient, making many tests extremely expensive. For example, an MRI (magnetic resonance imaging) scan, which lets your doctor "see" the details of tissues inside your body, costs $1,000 to $1,500 per test.

This expense may be worthwhile if the test leads to earlier diagnosis or better treatment of a serious problem. But you shouldn't assume that every test your doctor orders is likely to have that result. In fact, some tests may have the opposite effect, actually causing a delay in diagnosis or leading to the wrong therapy because the test was performed improperly and the results are inaccurate. Worse yet, some tests can cause side effects or complications that may even aggravate your medical condition. That's why it is so important to get only the tests you need, and only when they are likely to help you.

Questions to Ask Before You Have a Test

How can you tell which tests are really necessary? Here are six questions you should ask your physician the next time he or she recommends that a test be performed:

Refusing Tests: Art Ulene's Personal Experience

Not long ago, I was hospitalized for tests to determine why my blood sugar had dropped to a dangerous level on one occasion. One possible diagnosis my doctor was considering was a tumor in my pancreas, so he ordered an MRI (magnetic resonance imaging) scan of the pancreas. After reviewing the scan, the radiologist reported that it showed "possible enlargement of the pancreas," and recommended that I undergo a much more complicated procedure known as "retrograde endoscopic cannulation of the pancreatic duct" (it's done by passing a tube down through the mouth, stomach and small intestine, and then into the pancreas). I was very reluctant to have this test because there was a three percent chance that it would cause severe and long-lasting inflammation in my pancreas, not to mention its $2,000 price tag. To resolve the issue, I sent the scans to another radiologist for a second opinion—one who was very experienced in this particular area. He concluded that my pancreas was not enlarged and recommended against any further testing. Two problem-free years later, the decision to refuse that test looks even better.

• **Why is the test being ordered?**
Asking this question will help you
determine if the test is really necessary to diagnose your condition, or
if it is being ordered for a less justifiable reason.

> *Whatever your condition, don't
> be afraid to ask what new infor-
> mation is going to be gained
> from any test the doctor orders.*

You have a right to this information before you agree to undergo any
test. That right is called "informed consent." If your doctor doesn't
give you the information or can't give it to you in a way you can
understand, you should consider refusing the test and finding
another doctor.

• **What will the test reveal about my condition that is not already
known?** Some doctors order tests just to confirm what they already
know (long after your symptoms have passed, some of these doctors
are still ordering tests to prove that you are well). But, generally, you
shouldn't have to pay for tests that can't shed light on your condition. For example, if you've already taken a home pregnancy test and
a pelvic exam confirms that you are six weeks' pregnant, why pay for
an additional test in the doctor's office?

This is particularly important when the same test keeps getting repeated day after day. There are some times when repetitive testing can be
justified—for example, in people who are receiving cancer chemotherapy that could drop their blood counts down to dangerous levels.
But getting weekly blood tests makes no sense if you're being treated
for mild anemia and your therapy won't change no matter what the
test shows. Whatever your condition, don't be afraid to ask what new
information is going to be gained from any test the doctor orders.
Your doctor will either have a good answer, or you will have one less
test to undergo.

• **How will the test result change the way my case is managed?** Just
gathering information about your condition makes no sense if it isn't
going to change the way you are being treated.

That may seem obvious, but many tests are ordered without enough
attention to this point. People with terminal illnesses are probably the
biggest victims of this practice. Day after day, these poor souls are
jabbed for blood specimens and taken for x-rays when neither they

> *Studies show that doctors order fewer tests when they are reminded what the tests cost.*

nor their physicians have any intention of changing the basic treatment. You should not have any test—even one that will provide new information—unless the doctor can show you that the results could change the way you are treated.

• **What does the test cost?** This is one of the most important questions to ask if you want to save money. Studies show that doctors order fewer tests when they are reminded what the tests cost. This was neatly demonstrated in a study reported in *The New England Journal of Medicine.*

In this study, researchers observed the test-ordering behavior of doctors who worked on two different wards in the same hospital. Doctors on both wards used computer terminals to order tests on their patients, but on one ward, the computer was programmed to display on-screen the cost of each test whenever the doctor entered an order. On the other ward, the computer screen gave no indication of cost. The doctors who were continually reminded what each test cost ordered 14 percent fewer tests than did their colleagues who were unaware of these costs.

Some people are reluctant to ask questions about cost because they don't want to compromise the quality of their care over money. If that description fits you, let us remind you one more time that the quality of care is not related to how much money you spend, but how well you spend it. Spending too much money on the wrong tests will actually make the quality of your care go down.

• **What are the potential risks and side effects associated with the test itself?** Most people assume that tests are perfectly safe or doctors wouldn't order them. That's not a correct assumption because some tests have the potential for causing unpleasant—even dangerous—side effects or complications. It's worth accepting these risks when it is likely that the test will diagnose your problem or help your doctor treat you more effectively. But only you can decide whether you should take the risk or not. So, before you agree to have a test performed, learn everything you can about its possible side effects and complications. And don't forget to ask how often side effects and complications are likely to occur. A serious complication that occurs only one time in a million is probably not worth worrying about as much as a mildly disabling side effect that occurs ten percent of the time.

• **What alternatives are there to taking the test?** Most people are surprised to learn that there is often a good alternative when their doctor recommends that they take a test.

The simplest alternative, though not necessarily the wisest, is to skip the test. This is a good choice when the test is not really necessary or when its potential risks outweigh the potential benefits. Refusing a test is not a wise option, however, when doing so may delay diagnosis and treatment of a serious problem.

Sometimes, the wisest choice is the middle ground: delaying the test for a few hours (or days or weeks) to see if your medical problem resolves itself. Whenever your doctor recommends a test, it is perfectly reasonable to discuss this alternative. You should, however, be willing to have the test without delay if your doctor can make a persuasive argument for going ahead with it.

Often, you may have yet a third option: a different test that is less risky or less costly. Talking to your doctor is the best way to learn about this alternative, but it wouldn't hurt to do a little research yourself—especially if the recommended test is very complex or costly. You will find information about the most commonly performed tests in most medical encyclopedias and home health guides. Some of these books have charts that show you the order in which these tests should be done. Keep in mind that these charts are meant for general use, so the specific instructions may not be appropriate in your particular case. The best way to tell which information is relevant for you is to discuss what you have learned with your physician, and to ask questions.

A Resource Book on Testing

For a handy reference book on testing, consult the *Complete Guide to Medical Tests*, H. Winter Griffith, MD, Fisher Books, 1993. It describes hundreds of the most common medical tests, including risks, reliability and average costs; 932 pages, $17.95 (paperback).

Comparison Shopping

Once you know a test is necessary, you should have a strategy for cutting the costs of medical tests. Follow these steps to ensure you're getting the best price for any given test.

USE YOUR TELEPHONE TO COMPARE PRICES

As with other medical costs, such as physician fees and drugs, there can be a wide variation in the cost of tests within the same community. If you are willing to spend some time on the phone calling different facilities in your area, you may be able to save a significant amount of money on your medical test.

To demonstrate how much the price of tests can vary, we called a number of labs in the New Jersey and New York area to gather data

Cost Comparison for Blood Tests*

Test	Average Cost	Low–High Range
Complete Blood Count	$18.46	$13–$35
Quantitative Pregnancy	$52.71	$22–$84
Total Cholesterol	$18.76	$14–$33
Cholesterol Profile	$53.53	$38–$83

Cost Comparison of Radiological Tests*

Test	Average Cost	Low–High Range
CAT scan–head	$581.43	$400–$750
Ultrasound–OB	$226.00	$160–$325
Ultrasound–GI	$176.25	$150–$240
Ultrasound–Kidney	$181.25	$150–$240
Mammogram–baseline**	$124.87	$65–$180

*Source: Original research in the New York/New Jersey area
**You can receive a list of low-cost providers of mammography in your area by calling your local chapter of the American Cancer Society. Additionally, the ACS can advise you of upcoming free mammography screening clinics.

on costs for common blood tests. We also conducted a survey of different radiological (x-ray) tests for the same area of the country. The results of our survey are shown in the tables that appear on page 68. Our objective in listing these costs is to show you that it can really pay to "shop around"—even for medical tests.

DISCUSS TEST COSTS WITH YOUR PHYSICIAN

Your doctor will probably suggest where you should have a test done. Make sure your physician knows that cost is important to you. If the doctor can't assure you that the suggested testing facility charges low prices, do your own price-checking by phone before you go.

If You Are Going into the Hospital

Typically, outpatient testing is less expensive than inpatient testing. Complete as many of your preoperative tests as possible as an outpatient prior to checking into the hospital. Also, it is a waste of money to pay for a day in the hospital for testing when the same tests could be conducted as an outpatient. To give you an idea of the difference in costs, we compared the difference between inpatient rates at a community hospital and outpatient rates at a private clinic in the same area (see page 71).

Before you schedule any major test or medical procedure, it's a good idea to call your insurer (or ask your doctor to call) to determine whether your costs are best covered as an inpatient or an outpatient. Strange as it seems, some insurance plans are still requiring that you be hospitalized before they will pay for your procedures—even though this approach will probably cost them more money. Keep a record of your call, just in case the insurance company rejects payment of your bill.

BE SURE YOUR PREOPERATIVE TESTS ARE ESSENTIAL

Preoperative tests are used to detect underlying problems, which might affect a patient's operative or postoperative course. However, problems are detected infrequently as a result of these comprehensive tests. For example, a typical preoperative patient is usually put through the following tests:

CBC (complete blood count)	$ 13
SMAC (serum electrolytes)	$ 24
EKG (electrocardiogram)	$ 75
CXR (chest x-ray)	$100
U/A (urinalysis)	$ 14
Type and Hold (blood bank specimen)	$ 22
PT/PTT (clotting factor analysis)	$ 75
TOTAL	$323

Source: Original research

The above costs were quoted by a private, nonprofit, urban hospital in the northeast. Physicians typically order these tests by habit rather than by individual patient indications. So, like all other tests and therapies your physician recommends, always question each test to determine its usefulness and necessity.

A study reported in *JAMA: Journal of the American Medical Association* looked at the most commonly performed preoperative tests. The researchers found that the majority of preoperative tests performed were actually unnecessary, meaning that they added no new information to either diagnosis or treatment.

GET A SECOND OPINION BEFORE AGREEING TO COMPLEX, EXPENSIVE TESTS WITH HIGH RISKS

As with any medical procedure, if you have any doubt about a test's usefulness in your diagnosis or treatment, get a second opinion. In some cases, your insurance might pay for, or even require, a second opinion before it will cover the cost of an expensive procedure.

Avoid Unnecessary Duplication of Medical Tests

One of the easiest ways to save money on medical tests is to make sure that tests are not duplicated unnecessarily.

The best way to check this is to keep copies of all your medical test results. To do this, you must specifically ask for these results from your doctor and/or the lab. Additionally, whenever possible, keep original x-rays or other radiological films. If you have one primary physician, he or she can maintain all of these records for you and will send them on to any specialist that you may need to see. However, if you do not have an active relationship with a primary care provider, it is absolutely essential that you maintain your own records.

People with chronic conditions and the elderly are especially vulnerable to duplicate testing. They tend to see more specialists and to have many more tests. Even though you have a serious condition or a chronic disease, you must question each test and its validity.

NEVER PAY FOR TESTS THAT NEED TO BE REPEATED DUE TO CIRCUMSTANCES BEYOND YOUR CONTROL

On many occasions, tests must be repeated because someone has made a mistake. For example, you may need to have a blood test done and you must fast prior to the blood draw. Your doctor or his/her staff fail to instruct you not to eat on the test day. You do eat, so the test is invalid and must be repeated. You should not be charged for the second test.

Similarly, a physician schedules you for a CT scan. Technical problems prevent accurate imaging, so the test must be repeated. You should not have to pay for the second scan.

Or, say a lab misplaces your Pap smear. Your physician requests that you repeat the test. In this case, you should be charged only once for both the physician visit *and* the lab work. Take a hint from insurance companies. They will typically not pay for repetitive tests. You should follow their lead.

Cost Comparisons of Common Tests: Community Hospitals Versus Private Clinics*

Test	Community Hospital (inpatient)	Private Clinic (outpatient)
Echocardiogram	$913	$591
EKG	$ 93	$ 68
Blood Glucose	$ 37	$ 18

*Source: Original research

HOW TO SAVE MONEY ON MEDICATIONS

When carefully chosen and properly used, prescription and over-the-counter medications are among the best bargains in medical care today. They can be used to relieve symptoms, reduce suffering, eliminate the need for surgery and—in many cases—completely cure you of problems that range from minor to life-threatening.

But the same medications that are so helpful can have just the opposite effect if they are poorly selected or used inappropriately. In these situations, they can cause unpleasant and possibly dangerous side effects, sometimes even worsening the conditions they were meant to treat, and running up your medical expenses unnecessarily.

To Medicate or Not to Medicate?

Some people overuse medications. They "pop" pills at the drop of a hat. They take antibiotics for colds and medicate themselves to sleep. They use laxatives to deal with constipation and tranquilizers to cope with stress. They ignore the underlying causes of their problems and treat the symptoms instead. As a result, they waste a lot of money on medications that don't solve their real problems, while exposing themselves to the potential risks of these unnecessary medications.

Other people are at the opposite extreme: They simply refuse to take medications under almost any condition. This attitude makes no sense either medically or economically. Refusing to use antibiotics to treat an ear infection or a true "strep" throat may save a few dollars today, but invites disaster and high medical bills tomorrow because of the serious complications that can result.

> We think the best approach with both prescription and nonprescription medications is to use them whenever their cost and potential risks are outweighed by their potential benefits.

We think the best approach with both prescription and nonprescription medications is to use them whenever their cost and potential risks are outweighed by their potential benefits. In other words, medications make sense when there is a high probability they will be effective for treating your medical problem, a low probability they will cause unpleasant or dangerous side effects, and the cost is reasonable for the benefits you could get from them.

Unfortunately, it is very difficult (even for your physician) to accurately and objectively measure the risks and benefits of many medications, and even more difficult to balance the risks and benefits against each other. For example, there are some extraordinary potential benefits for women who take estrogen after menopause: In addition to eliminating hot flashes, estrogen dramatically reduces the occurrence of bone fractures in women who are at risk for osteoporosis, and it reduces the incidence of heart attacks (by as much as 50 percent) in women who are at risk for coronary heart disease. But women who take estrogen have an increased risk of developing uterine cancer, and they may have a very slightly increased risk of developing breast cancer. The woman who has several family members with breast cancer and none with osteoporosis may find these risks too worrisome. But a woman at high risk for osteoporosis and heart disease may find estrogen replacement therapy very appealing.

Another thing that makes decisions about medications difficult is that you never know which side effects and benefits you'll end up getting until after you take the medication. If a medication works well and you get no bad side effects from taking it, you're a winner. But how will you feel if the medication doesn't work and it causes you to have a major allergic reaction? Not very happy, but—by then—it's too late to take back your decision to use the medication.

In that sense, your decisions about medications are like all your other decisions in life. You never really know how they're going to turn out until you put them into action, but you still want to make as intelligent decisions as possible.

The box below offers some basic rules to follow when taking medications. These guidelines seem so simple and obvious, you would think that everyone already follows them. In reality, most people take whatever medications their doctors order without asking about risks and benefits, and without inquiring about alternatives. These same people buy their medications at the most convenient location, without any consideration of price. As if that weren't enough, studies show that the majority of people who are given prescriptions do not take their medications properly. As a result, they expose themselves to unnecessary medical risks and waste huge sums of money. In the rest of this chapter, we'll show you how you can help avoid these problems by learning to ask the right questions.

Balancing Risks and Benefits

Any medication that is powerful enough to do some good in your body is also powerful enough to cause unpleasant—even dangerous—side effects. Sometimes, the side effects must be tolerated because the disease for which the medication is prescribed is so serious (as in the case of chemotherapy for cancer). But there are times when the potential risks of using medications outweigh their potential benefits—for example, taking a medication with potentially dangerous side effects to treat a minor illness that will go away by itself. Yet

Medication Guidelines

Here are some simple guidelines that will help you get the most benefit from medications:

- Use medications only when the potential benefits are greater than the potential risks.

- Whenever a medication is recommended by your physician, make sure it is the best alternative among all of the therapies available for treating your particular condition.

- Buy all of your medications at the lowest practical price.

- Use all medications properly.

> *Most people take whatever medications their doctors order without asking about risks and benefits.*

millions of Americans do just that every year when they use antibiotics to treat colds and flu. Everyone knows that antibiotics don't kill the viruses that cause colds and flu, but that does not stop some doctors from prescribing them. Patients who are treated this way leave the doctor's office with prescriptions they don't need and with greater risks of medical problems because of the unnecessary medications.

Other people make just the opposite mistake, by refusing to take recommended medications when the potential benefits far outweigh the risks. There is nothing more tragic than seeing a minor infection turn into a life-threatening illness because a patient refused to take antibiotics when they were really needed, or watching people suffer strokes because they refused to take medication for high blood pressure. We have seen this happen again and again.

Many people assume that their physicians will prescribe medications only when the potential benefits outweigh the risks. But some doctors admit that they routinely write prescriptions to justify the cost of an office visit. (Strange as it sounds, many patients feel cheated if they are charged for a visit where nothing wrong is found and no prescription is written.) Other physicians tell us that some patients literally demand medications in situations where they are not likely to benefit (for example, to treat the flu). Too often, the doctors prescribe medications to avoid a battle or because they know the patient will simply go see another physician who is willing to write the prescription. Whatever the reason, 60 percent of all visits to a physician result in some type of medication therapy.

Another problem that can make it harder to decide about medications is that many doctors are simply not familiar with all of the risks and benefits for every medication they prescribe. There are literally thousands of medications available today, each with its own long list of special warnings. It's almost impossible for a doctor to keep up with all of these medications, not to mention all of the new medications coming to market every year. And few doctors take enough time to explain everything a patient needs to know about a medication before using it.

So how can you decide whether to take a medication or not? There is no precise formula for balancing the benefits of a medication against the risks of side effects and the medication's cost. But common sense tells us that you will make better decisions when you take these factors into consideration than when you blindly accept or reject a prescription on your intuition. The key to making an intelligent decision is to get as much information as possible about the treatment you are considering.

> *There is nothing more tragic than seeing a minor infection turn into a life-threatening illness because a patient refused to take antibiotics when they were really needed.*

Making Sure Medication Is the Best Alternative

Many people are taking medications for colds and flu when they could be treated just as well—or better—without them. Using antibiotics may be justifiable in selected patients with serious medical disorders (such as cystic fibrosis or chronic heart or lung disease) that increase their risk of developing pneumonia or other complications while sick with influenza. But every year, millions of Americans at low risk for such complications are paying for antibiotics that cannot benefit them in any way, but which expose them needlessly to the risk of side effects. These people should have been told that they would get over their colds without any treatment other than the rest and nutrition needed to promote recovery.

The abuse of medications is not limited to antibiotics for colds. Millions of doses of sleeping pills are prescribed every year for chronic insomnia, when counseling and relaxation techniques would be a better choice. Cholesterol-lowering medications are used in place of serious dietary changes; appetite suppressant medications instead of sensible diets and exercise; and high blood pressure pills instead of salt restriction and weight loss.

The final decision about which medications you will take is up to you, and that's the way it should be. After all, you are the one who will take the risks and pay the bills, and you are the one who will receive the benefits. It's only right that you decide whether the potential benefits justify the potential risks in your case. To make good decisions, you will need a lot of information, and you will probably have to ask a lot of questions.

There are some questions that only your doctor can answer when a medication is prescribed (for example, questions about your diagnosis, the reason a particular medication was selected, and what other alternatives are available). Use the Medication Questionnaire on page 80 as a guide to which questions to ask. Many other questions (such as what foods, if any, need to be avoided while taking the medication) can be answered just as well—or better—by your pharmacist or by checking a reliable reference book about medications.

Getting answers to all of these questions may sound like a lot of work, and you may think it's really your doctor's and pharmacist's responsibility to worry about these things, but if you leave it entirely up to them you could be taking unnecessary risks and wasting money.

Our advice is simple: Don't start any new medication until you are satisfied that the potential benefits outweigh the potential risks, and until you have explored all other appropriate alternatives (we emphasize the word "appropriate" because there are almost always some alternatives available that make no medical sense).

The Potential Cost of Refusing Medication

CONSIDER THE COST OF NOT USING MEDICATIONS TO TREAT CERTAIN MEDICAL PROBLEMS:

- The price of not treating severe hypertension (high blood pressure) is an increased risk of heart attack, stroke and kidney failure.

- Not treating an ulcer increases your risk of gastrointestinal bleeding and anemia, which means there's a greater chance you'll need an operation to treat the problem.

- The penalty for refusing to use cholesterol-lowering medications when dietary measures don't work is an increased risk of heart attack and stroke.

- Not treating severe depression increases the risk of suicide.

NON-DRUG ALTERNATIVES

Perhaps the best way to save money on medications is to use non-drug alternatives when they are appropriate. If your problem is a mild case of elevated blood cholesterol, dietary changes may be the best way to manage it (by decreasing your intake of cholesterol and fat—especially saturated fat). Not everyone responds to diet alone, but for those who do, it's a simple, safe and very inexpensive alternative to cholesterol-lowering medications.

Here are a few more examples of medical problems that often lend themselves to nonmedical solutions:

Smoking Cessation: Nicotine patches can be very helpful if you are nicotine-addicted and you want to quit smoking. The patches help prevent withdrawal symptoms, and they double the success rate for nicotine addicts. But more than 60 percent of smokers are not addicted to nicotine, so the patch is of little or no value to them. For these people, a suggested ten-week prescription for patches costs over $300, but adds essentially nothing to their success rate. Millions of us have quit smoking without the patch.

Weight Loss: Without question, using medications to treat weight loss is one of the most controversial areas of medicine. In part, that's because the medications that were commonly used for this purpose twenty to thirty years ago turned out either to be worthless (HCG hormone injections) or dangerously addictive (amphetamine drugs, often referred to as "uppers"). Today, other appetite-suppressing drugs are available that promote weight loss without the danger of addiction. However, use of these medications is still accompanied by significant side effects in a large percentage of cases, and research shows that the overwhelming majority of people gain their weight right back again as soon as they stop using the medications.

We do not want to minimize the difficulty many people have controlling their weight, but we cannot justify the risks of using drugs to treat this problem. Instead, we recommend that this problem be managed through dietary changes (primarily by eliminating fat as much as possible from your diet) and regular physical activity (just walking at a brisk pace for twenty minutes every day will suffice).

Medication Questionnaire

The following list contains questions to ask about every medication you use before you start taking it. Your physician is the best source for this information, but your doctor may be too busy to cover all of the questions or may not know the answers to all of them. You can also get answers to many questions from your pharmacist or a good reference book on drugs, such as *The American Medical Association Guide to Prescription and Over-the-Counter Drugs*. At the very least, you should discuss with your physician the following questions:

- What condition is this medication being prescribed for?
- How will this medication help me, and what is the likelihood that it will actually cure my illness or get rid of my symptoms?
- How does the medication work?
- How long will I have to take the medication?
- What are the side effects of this medication, and what risks am I taking by using it? What should I do if I experience any side effects?
- What are the alternatives to taking the medication:

  Are there any other medications that are more likely to work or less likely to cause side effects or that are less expensive?

  Are there other treatments for my condition that do not involve medications?

  What is the risk of simply waiting and watching—without any treatment—to see if I get better by myself?

- Is there a generic version of the medication available or another brand that would cost less money? Is the generic version really equivalent to the name brand?
- How and when should the medication be taken?
- Are there any foods, beverages, or activities that must be avoided while using the medication?
- Do you have any samples of this medication for me to try out before I fill the prescription?

If you don't have answers to all of the questions above for the medications you are taking, then you really don't have the information you need to make an intelligent decision about whether or not you should be taking them.

Chronic Back Pain: The overwhelming majority of back pain is due to poor physical conditioning, improper use of the back, and stress (stress causes chronic tension in the back muscles, which produces the pain). When the problem is caused by an acute injury, the use of pain medication and muscle-relaxing medications may be appropriate *for a short period of time.* However, the use of medications (especially ones that are potentially addicting) cannot be justified for the treatment of chronic pain. In some cases, the long-term solution to this problem is an exercise program to recondition the muscles, instruction on how to use the back properly, and a stress management program.

Coronary Artery Disease: This condition is the leading cause of death in both men and women (it strikes women a little later in life, but no less often). The medical approach to coronary heart disease uses medications to control blood pressure, lower blood cholesterol, promote smoking cessation and weight loss, and reduce symptoms related to stress. When these methods fail, invasive procedures such as angioplasty or coronary bypass surgery are often used. The natural approach uses diet, exercise, deep relaxation techniques, and education to lower cholesterol, blood pressure and stress levels. For some people, the natural approach will prevent—even reverse—atherosclerosis. Others, particularly those who have hereditary problems leading to their high blood cholesterol levels, may need medications, as well.

Getting the Best Medication

When your doctor prescribes a medication for you, it's natural to assume that he or she picked the best medication for your specific problem. But don't bet your life on that assumption, because choosing the right medication for a medical problem is part science, part art and part luck.

There are many reasons why you could get the wrong medication. In fairness to the doctors who treat you, we must point out that picking the right medication is not always as simple as it sounds. There are more than 3,000 medications currently available, and every year approximately 25 new drugs are brought on the market.

To cope with this overwhelming list of medications many physicians try to become very familiar with one or two drugs in each major category, and then pretty much limit themselves to using those. For example, to treat patients with high blood pressure (a category for which the latest *Physician's Desk Reference* lists almost 100 different choices), many doctors will rely on one medication from each of five chemically different groups, and use the one that seems best-suited to a particular patient. Other doctors will start all hypertensive patients on the same medication, no matter what their medical condition, switching to other medications only if the first one doesn't work. The difference in cost, depending on which strategy your doctor chooses and which medication he or she selects from each category, could amount to hundreds of dollars per year.

Some physicians will continue to prescribe the same drug for years— or even decades—even after more effective or less expensive alternatives become available. After using one medication for a long time, it's easy for a doctor to become very comfortable with it. That makes it difficult to switch to a new medication that works differently.

THE DRUG COMPANIES' ROLE

The pharmaceutical companies have invested huge sums of money developing medications and so put a great deal of effort into promoting these medications to doctors. For example, there are nearly 20 different nonsteroidal anti-inflammatory medications (not counting aspirin) for treating arthritis. The pharmaceutical companies would like doctors (and you) to believe that each of these medications is unique, while the chemical differences between them often don't translate into significant clinical differences in your body.

In most industries, competition between similar products would have resulted in dramatic price drops. That has not been the case with pharmaceuticals. But now, as we enter the era of "managed competition," some drug companies are beginning to compete by reducing their prices. This means that you may now be able to save some money by asking your doctor to switch you to a lower-priced brand in the same group of medications.

Some prescription and over-the-counter medications truly are unique, like clozapine (used to treat schizophrenia) or sumatriptan (used to treat migraine headaches). If you have one of those disorders, your doctor may feel that there is no other appropriate alternative to these medications. But these situations are rare. Much more often, your doctor will be able to choose from several medications that are equally effective for treating your condition. In that case, you want to be sure that your doctor has prescribed (or, in the case of nonprescription medications, that you have chosen) the least expensive medication.

The "Comparing Medications" chart on page 86 lists several medication categories in which all of the drugs in that group are chemically

Why Isn't the Non-Medication Approach More Popular?

If the natural, non-medicated approach is so effective, why don't all doctors use it? Here are a few reasons we've heard to explain this disappointing situation:

- **Doctors receive little training in the natural approach.** Most of their education takes place in hospital settings with sick patients who require medical treatments. As medical students, they are overwhelmed with information about every disease. But they receive relatively little information about basic issues such as nutrition, exercise, stress management and alternatives to medical therapies.

- **Doctors are not paid well for using the natural approach.** By and large, doctors get paid for doing things to people, not for talking to them. That's why surgeons and other specialists make so much more than family physicians and pediatricians. And that's why it's so difficult to get some doctors interested in the natural approach to healing. It takes much longer to teach a patient about a cholesterol-lowering diet than it does to prescribe a cholesterol-lowering medication, and no one is willing to pay for that extra time.

- **Many physicians believe that the natural approach doesn't work.** After seeing countless patients smoke, avoid exercise, gain weight and drink to excess, many physicians have simply given up on the natural approach in the sincere belief that it doesn't work. The truth is, it doesn't work for some people. But neither do many of the medications and other treatments that doctors prescribe. So your best bet is to find a physician who's willing to try natural methods first, when they are appropriate.

> Some physicians will continue to prescribe the same drug for years—even after more effective or less expensive alternatives become available.

similar and produce similar results. There may be some slight differences among the medications within each group, but more often than not, these differences have not been proven to be clinically meaningful. You should ask your doctor to prescribe the least expensive one whenever possible. Your doctor should have no objection to using the least expensive medication in the group.

As the chart illustrates, there are some very big price differences between medications in the same category. These price differences become even more significant if you will be taking the medication every day for the rest of your life. While you should always ask your doctor to choose the lowest-price option when possible, your doctor may have an important medical reason for choosing a more expensive medication in the category. If so, learning that reason will make you feel better about paying the difference.

Oral contraceptives are a good example of a group of medications where the differences between the brands may not make a difference in your body, but can affect the price you are charged. During the last decade, several so-called "tricyclic" birth control pills have been introduced, and manufacturers have spent tens of millions of dollars (perhaps hundreds of millions) to create the impression that these pills are better than the old ones.

However, tricyclic pills are no more effective at preventing pregnancy, they are no safer, and they have just as many (or as few) side effects as the old pills. So, when getting a prescription for birth control pills, be sure your doctor doesn't simply prescribe the newest pill for you. Instead, discuss all the available options that fit your needs—both medically and financially.

Shop Around for Your Medications

The price of medications can vary tremendously depending on where you buy them, which form of a medication you choose, and the quantity purchased. Pharmacies can legally charge whatever they want for medications, so some pharmacies (not many) charge whatever the traffic will bear. Others choose exactly the opposite approach. Some chains and discount stores use prescription medications as "loss leaders"—they literally sell some medications below their own cost to get customers into the stores, where they can sell other profitable products to them. Most pharmacies select the middle ground, charging just enough to cover the cost of the medications and the store's overhead while allowing for a fair profit.

Most people are surprised to learn how much extra money they may spend by choosing the wrong pharmacy for their medications. In a comparison test, we found a pharmacy that was charging three times as much for the same medication as a drugstore that was virtually across the street. While this case represented an extreme example of price gouging, it is not unusual to find some pharmacies charging 40 percent to 50 percent more than other pharmacies in the same city for the same medications. How can pharmacies get away with this? Very easily, if you let them.

BUY AT THE LOWEST PRACTICAL PRICE

Our advice is simple: Buy your medications at the lowest *practical* price. We'd like to say you should buy medications at the lowest *possible* price, but there are times when this is not the smartest thing to do. For example, it's not worth driving 20 miles across town to save two dollars on a prescription you'll only fill once, because it will cost more than two dollars in gas and time. And if you've got an ear infection that needs treatment today, it's not sensible to order antibiotics by mail, even if you could save $15, because your ear could be ruined by the infection before the antibiotics arrive.

But there are many times when it does pay to go the extra distance or to use a mail-order pharmacy instead of the drugstore around the corner. For example, a mail-order pharmacy might save you 19 cents per pill compared to a local independent pharmacy. If you were taking medication twice a day, this adds up to a savings of $138.70 at the end of a year. And a 20 percent to 30 percent discount on your daily cholesterol-lowering medication, when purchased at a chain discount pharmacy or through mail order, could save you more than $400 a year.

Comparing Medications

To give you an idea of how much you could save by asking your doctor for the least expensive medication, look at the chart below, which lists comparative prices for groups of medications used to treat ulcers, high blood pressure, high cholesterol, depression and arthritis.

We priced the following medications at a large chain pharmacy. In all cases, the medications we compared were for chronic conditions and for a one-month supply. These prescription drugs were compared at therapeutically equivalent dosages.

ULCER MEDICATIONS
Prilosec–$113.25	Zantac–$98.70
Carafate–$90.30	Tagamet–$88.15

HIGH BLOOD PRESSURE MEDICATIONS
Vasotec–$67.60	Lotension–$45.25
Capoten–$43.55	Monopril–$31.40

CHOLESTEROL-LOWERING AGENTS
Pravachol–$64.60	Zocor–$58.45
Mevacor–$52.10	

ANTIDEPRESSANTS
Prozac–$79.50	Paxil–$73.20
Zoloft–$61.05	

PAIN MEDICATIONS (Nonsteroidal anti-inflammatory agents)
Naprosyn–$77.55	Anaprox–$77.30
Tolectin (brand tolmetin sodium)–$104.35	
Generic (tolmetin sodium)–$74.00	
Motrin (brand ibuprofen)–$39.95	
Generic (ibuprofen)–$22.00	

Please note that while there are several medications listed for each class, there may be subtle differences between the medications, and a more expensive medication may be the best choice for you in some cases. You should ask your physician to prescribe the lowest price medication whenever it does not make a difference clinically.

SELECT THE LOWEST-PRICED PRODUCT

Sometimes, the medications your doctor can choose from will not only be chemically similar—they will be chemically identical. This happens because some pharmaceutical companies are now licensing their new medications to other companies. The two companies use different brand-names for the same medication and then spend millions of advertising dollars to persuade physicians to prescribe their brand. A good

> *We found a pharmacy that was charging three times as much for the same medication as a drugstore that was virtually across the street.*

example of this is lisinopril (used to treat high blood pressure). Merck Sharp & Dohme, the developer of lisinopril, markets the medication under the brand-name "Prinivil." But Stuart Pharmaceuticals markets the identical drug under the brand-name "Zestril." Medical journals are filled with ads designed to convince doctors of the superiority of one brand or the other (although, since they are chemically identical, it's not possible for one to be superior to the other).

Why would drug companies compete with themselves? Because the company that develops the new medication gets a share of the second company's sales, and the second company gets a new product to market without risking hundreds of millions of dollars on new drug development. Both companies make higher profits because their investment and risk are reduced, while you pay higher prices to cover the doubled cost of marketing.

Theoretically, the competition should result in lower prices. But the drug companies haven't tried to compete this way. Still, it does pay to shop around if you know that another, identical brand exists (we'll show you how to determine that in a moment). We priced both brands of lisinopril at a chain drugstore in Los Angeles, and found

PRICE DIFFERENCE BY BRAND FOR LISINOPRIL

Prinivil (Merck Sharp & Dohme)	20 mg 100 tabs	$91.30
Zestril (Stuart Pharmaceuticals)	20 mg 100 tabs	$98.35

differences of as much as $7.05 per 100 tablets. That may not sound like much until you consider the fact that some people with hypertension may use this medication for years.

GENERIC DRUGS VS. BRAND-NAMES

Sometimes, drug companies don't have a choice about the competition. Once a company's patent protection runs out on a medication it has developed, other companies are legally entitled to copy the medication and produce it themselves. These copies, known as "generic drugs," are then sold in competition with the original brands, but often at much lower prices.

Usually—but not always—a generic drug is your best buy. The FDA requires that the active medication in a generic drug be chemically identical to the brand that is being copied. But generic drugs can vary from the original brand in other respects: They may contain different fillers, binders, coatings, colorings and preservatives, so it's possible for them to react a little differently in your body.

The FDA permits a generic drug to differ up to 20 percent from the original brand in the rate at which the medication is absorbed into your bloodstream (either faster or slower). Under most circumstances, this is not enough to make a real difference in the results you will get from the medication, and it's not likely to cause trouble if your doctor prescribes the generic drug from the very beginning of your therapy. However, problems can arise if you are switching from the brand-name version of a medication to a generic, or vice versa. With some medications, such as anticonvulsants for epilepsy and medications for heart problems, a difference of 20 percent more or less in your bloodstream could have some effect, so any symptoms that arise after switching must be reported promptly to your physician. Children and older people are generally more sensitive to changes in their medications, so switches from brand-name medications to generics (or vice versa) should be made carefully in these groups.

You can save money without sacrificing your health by asking your doctor to prescribe a generic whenever possible, and then asking your pharmacist to assure you that the generic is really equivalent to the brand-name version. If your pharmacist has any concern about the generic version, he or she will recommend that you remain with the brand-name version.

OVER-THE-COUNTER MEDICATIONS

Some prescription medications are also available in a chemically identical over-the-counter version. The only difference is in the dose—the nonprescription product will usually have a dose that is lower than the prescription form. This difference can easily be overcome by taking two or three nonprescription pills instead of one of prescription-strength.

> *Some prescription medications are also available in a chemically identical over-the-counter version. The only difference is in the dose—the nonprescription product will usually have a dose that is lower than the prescription form.*

One example of a popular medication that is available in both prescription and nonprescription forms is Tavist, an antihistamine and decongestant. The nonprescription form, called Tavist-D, is half the strength of the prescription brand. Here are the prices a local pharmacy quoted to us:

Tavist-D (over-the-counter) 1.34 mg: 32 tablets $15

Tavist (prescription) 2.68 mg: 16 tablets $22

Thirty-two tablets of Tavist-D are equivalent to 16 tablets of Tavist. In this case, using the nonprescription version would save you $7 over the prescription brand.

The same rules apply to a commonly used antihistamine with the chemical name of diphenhydramine (you probably know it better by its brand-name: Benadryl). Look at the difference in price between the prescription form of this medication and the generic over-the-counter version. Ironically, you'd end up paying more for the brand-name version over-the-counter than for a prescription if you really needed the 50 milligram dose.

Benadryl (over-the-counter) 25 mg: 96 tablets $11.90

Generic (over-the-counter) 25 mg: 100 tablets $3.50

Benadryl (prescription) 50 mg: 48 tablets $14.65

Another good example is the drug ibuprofen, which is widely used to treat arthritis, menstrual cramps, and other aches and pains. Originally, ibuprofen was only available as the brand-name prescription drug Motrin. But now its patent has expired, and it has been released in a lower-dose nonprescription form that is widely available (ibuprofen is the medicine in Nuprin, Advil and several other brands). If your doctor thinks you should take ibuprofen, you can get it in any one of the following ways:

- Your doctor can prescribe Motrin (they are still selling this brand in 300 to 800 milligram strengths).

- Your doctor can prescribe generic ibuprofen (your pharmacist will probably fill the prescription with a generic copy of Motrin).

- Your doctor can tell you that you need ibuprofen and recommend that you ask your pharmacist to fill it in the cheapest manner possible, which will probably be an over-the-counter version of the medication.

The choice your doctor makes can have a significant effect on the price you end up paying. Here's what we found when we compared prices for the three choices listed above.

- If you filled a prescription for 100 tablets (800 milligram strength) of Motrin, the price would be $39.95.

- If you filled a prescription for generic ibuprofen (also 800 milligram strength), the price would be $22.00.

- If you purchased 400 tablets of the name brands (Advil or Nuprin) without a prescription (the nonprescription versions of ibuprofen only come in 200 milligram strength) and then took four tablets at each dose to get your 800 milligrams (200 mg x 4 pills = 800 mg), your total cost would be $36.00. Surprise! Here's a situation where the over-the-counter drug costs more than one of the prescription versions. But if your doctor had prescribed only 400 milligrams per dose, the nonprescription form might have come out better.

- If you purchased 400 tablets of the generic nonprescription form of ibuprofen (200 milligrams each) and took four tablets at each dose, your total cost would be $28.00. (Surprise, again! This is still more expensive than getting a prescription for the generic 800 milligram tablets.)

Your doctor should let you know you whenever a prescribed medication is also available without a prescription. This will give you a chance to compare prices and will sometimes result in a lower price for you (the savings with some drugs can amount to 50 percent or more). Some doctors fail to do this, either because of insensitivity to your financial concerns or because they believe that writing the prescription will make a more powerful impression on you. This is sheer nonsense!

Another possible exception to the rule of using over-the-counter versions of a medication is when your insurance will only cover prescription medications. In that situation, you may wish to get the prescription filled, but ask the pharmacist to select the lowest-priced version of the drug available.

Things to Consider When Choosing a Pharmacy

When choosing a place to buy your medications, price is an important factor, but not the only one. Here are some other issues you should consider when making your selection:

• **Availability of the pharmacist for counseling:** Next to your doctor, the best place to get information about your medications is directly from the pharmacist. (In fact, pharmacists are required by law to counsel their customers about every medication they dispense.) But it's not always easy to talk to the pharmacist; indeed, some busy pharmacies deliberately make it difficult to communicate with a pharmacist because it costs the store so much to provide this service. When choosing a pharmacy, realize that the most valuable product your pharmacy has to offer is not a medication (you can get that anywhere) but the information you need to use the medication properly and to avoid dangerous side effects.

• **Maintenance of patient profiles:** Some medications can produce dangerous reactions when taken at the same time as other medications. A very dramatic example of this occurred in early 1993, when several patients who were taking prescription antihistamines and antifungal medications—neither of which caused problems alone—suffered severe reactions when the two medications were taken together. Several people actually died from these reactions.

Next to your doctor, the best place to get information about your medications is directly from the pharmacist.

Ordinarily, your physician will try to avoid dangerous drug combinations. But if you are seeing more than one physician, and each doctor is prescribing medications without knowing what the other has already ordered, it's possible to get two prescriptions that don't mix safely.

The best way to avoid this problem is by patronizing one pharmacist who keeps track of all your medications (including over-the-counter medications) and who checks to be sure there are no dangerous combinations. Many pharmacists maintain a written record for each client, but more and more, the process is being computerized. Every time a new prescription is entered into the system, the computer automatically checks it against all of the other medications you are taking and against a database that contains all of the known interactions between medications. Whatever the method used, this is an essential service that could prevent you from suffering a dangerous drug reaction. Make sure you get this service when you buy medications.

If you use more than one pharmacy, you need to inform each pharmacist of all medications you are taking (including over-the-counter medications), no matter where you buy them. Don't be embarrassed about admitting that you buy some medications elsewhere. This is the only way the pharmacist can protect you against dangerous drug interactions. To accomplish this, you need to keep a list of your prescriptions. Or you can keep the pharmacy receipts for all your prescriptions and show them to any pharmacist filling a new prescription for you. In fact, this may be an opportunity to ask the pharmacist to match or even better your best price on all your prescriptions.

• **Convenience (location and hours of service):** This is an obvious factor to consider in your choice of a pharmacy, but you will have to balance convenience against the potential price you will pay for it. The hours of service can also be very important, since there may be occasions when you will need to get a prescription filled at night or on a Sunday. You should select a pharmacy that has made arrangements for emergency prescriptions during these hours (many pharmacists take calls from home).

If you choose a pharmacy that is open 24 hours a day, 7 days a week, be prepared to spend a little more for your prescriptions. This is not something to complain about—it costs a lot of money to keep a pharmacist on the premises around-the-clock.

• **Ancillary services:** Expect to pay extra for services such as delivery of medications to your home. In some cases, it may be worth the extra charge. If your pharmacy delivers medications without adding an extra charge, you can assume that it's built into the price of the medications. In this case, if you choose to pick up the prescriptions yourself, you should ask the pharmacist to deduct something from the price you pay to make up for the delivery costs that the store will save.

• **Pricing Policy:** The easiest way to save money on the medications you buy is to shop for the lowest price. Some stores will actually sell medications at a loss in order to entice customers into the store.

It's important to note that a pharmacy's medication prices do not stay the same, even on a week-to-week basis. Just because a pharmacy was the lowest at one time does not mean it will stay the lowest. In fact, we talked to the owner of an independent pharmacy who said he would match the lowest price available anytime a customer asked him to, rather than lose the customer. He also pointed out that he's on call from home on nights and weekends when the large chain stores are closed and their pharmacists are nowhere to be found. Finally, notice the good prices offered through mail order. For on-going medications or those that are not needed immediately, mail order is an excellent way to "shop." Let's look at how mail order works.

Mail-Order Pharmacies

If you are taking any medications for long periods of time (for example, blood pressure medications, cholesterol-lowering medications, estrogen), you may get your greatest savings by using a mail-order pharmacy. Although perhaps not appropriate for those in need of a short-term, one-time prescription, if you have been given an expensive, long-term prescription, you should definitely investigate the cost of buying your medication by mail. Many large and medium-size corporations have contracted with mail-order pharmacies for their employees. Also, many unions or service organizations (like the

If you are taking any medications for long periods of time, you may get your greatest savings by using a mail-order pharmacy.

Lion's Club) and other groups providing a third-party payer insurance plan probably have contracted with a mail order pharmacy.

The services listed below are open to the public; note that there can be significant price variations even among the mail-order pharmacies.

Action Mail Order Drug—(800) 452-1976
P.O. Box 787
Waterville, ME 04903

Call the above number for a price quote on your prescription and to place your order. You can pay via credit card or prepay by sending in a check. Then, have your doctor call in the prescription at the same number. There is no shipping charge for orders up to three pounds. This company also offers over-the-counter medications.

Medi-Mail/Mail Rx—(800) 331-1458
871-C Grier Drive
Las Vegas, NV 89119

To place an order, call with the full name of your prescribing physician, complete address, phone number, and prescription name and dosage. The company will verify all this information with your physician and then process your order. You may pay by credit card or send a check, which must be received before your medication can be sent. All orders, regardless of size, will have a postage and handling fee added. Orders arrive in 7 to 14 days.

The American Association of Retired Persons (AARP)
For Prices and Initial Orders: (800) 456-2226
For Refills on Prescriptions: (800) 456-2277

Pharmacy Service
144 Freeman Bridge Road
P.O. Box 2211
Schenectady, NY 12301-2211

To place an order, call AARP with the name of the prescription, name and phone number of the prescribing doctor, and your name, address, phone number, and birth date. Shipping charges on all orders, regardless of size, is $1.00. You should receive your shipment in about seven days.

Cystic Fibrosis Foundation Pharmacy Services—(800) 541-4959
CFF Home Health & Pharmacy Services
6931 Arlington Road, Suite T-200
Bethesda, MD 20814-9650

The CFF Pharmacy carries more than 150 medications, including enzyme supplements, antibiotics, aerosol medications, and some vitamins, to meet the needs of all individuals with cystic fibrosis. The CFF Pharmacy is able to offer many medications at costs lower than wholesale. This pharmacy will accept most insurance prescription drug cards.

Medications Resource Books

The standard book on medications used by doctors is the *Physician's Desk Reference* or "PDR." This book is available in libraries and bookstores, and contains reprints of the prescribing information that is approved by the FDA and that drug companies must provide to physicians. For the average consumer, the PDR is difficult to read and hard to understand. It also costs about $50.00. While this is an important reference book for physicians, we do not recommend it for consumers. Instead, we suggest any of the following books, written specifically for consumers, that are available for a significantly lower price. Because new medications are introduced every year, the latest books will be the most inclusive. In most cases, these books are also available at your public library.

The Essential Guide to Prescription Drugs 1993 by James W. Long, M.D. HarperPerennial, 1993, 1100 pages, $16.00.

Provides detailed information on the most prescribed medications and most used nonprescription medications; includes extensive discussion of drug therapy for chronic conditions. Written in a fairly technical style.

The Complete Drug Reference. U.S. Pharmacopeia Convention. Consumer Reports Books, 1993, 1713 pages, $39.95.

Straightforward information on currently marketed prescription and over-the-counter medications written in language aimed at the consumer.

Guide To Shopping for Your Medications

Once you and your doctor have decided that a medication is the best way to treat a condition, you must now decide how to get the medication in the least expensive, most efficient manner.

If the medication is a prescription that you need immediately:

- Gather all your medication information:
    - Brand-name of medication
    - Generic name of medication
    - Dosage
    - Number of refills
    - Insurance information
- Call a national chain discount store with a pharmacy in your area (such as Wal-Mart, Thrifty, CVS, Sav-On/Osco, etc.).
- Ask if they have the necessary medication in stock and get a price for it at the prescribed dosage.
- Call your most convenient pharmacy and check the price there. Make sure the store will honor any insurance drug program you have.
- Ask if they offer a discount for senior citizens, if applicable.
- If you would prefer to patronize your local pharmacy, ask them if they can match or come close to the lowest price you've found, or if they would be willing to give you a discount for filling all refills with them.
- Have your physician call in the prescription at the store you have chosen. Calling it in ahead will minimize your wait when you go to pick up the prescription.
- Be sure you get all your insurance receipts when you pick up your prescription.
- Request that the pharmacist enter this prescription and any others you may be taking, including over-the-counter medicines, in your "patient profile."
- Take your medication as prescribed.
- If you will need to refill the medicine, call a mail-order pharmacy and check the price. If it is lower than your local pharmacy, have your physician call in your next prescription now so that it will be delivered by the time your current prescription lapses. (Some mail-order companies will call the doctor for you.) As mail order is typically the least expensive way to purchase medications, it is ideal for medications that you need on a regular basis. Talk with the mail-order company you choose about its program for regular prescription refills.

The Pill Book. Bantam Books, 1992, 1016 pages, $6.99 (paperback).

Basically a layperson's translation of *The Physician's Desk Reference*; an easy-to-use reference guide. Illustrated.

Complete Guide to Prescription & Nonprescription Drugs by H. Winter Griffith. The Body Press, 1991, $15.95 (paperback).

A good guide for basic information on commonly used medications.

AARP Pharmacy Service Prescription Drug Handbook. American Association of Retired Persons, 1992, $12.95.

Organized by specific medical conditions with explanations as to why a medication is prescribed and what other medications are available. This reference book is developed especially for older persons. Illustrated.

The American Medical Association Guide to Prescription and Over-the-Counter Drugs. Random House, Inc., 1990, $25.00.

Covers commonly prescribed and widely used over-the-counter medications in clear and nontechnical language. Illustrated.

FREE DRUG PROGRAMS FOR PEOPLE IN NEED

Over 50 pharmaceutical manufacturers offer free medication programs to people who wouldn't otherwise be able to afford medications or for whom purchase would create a financial hardship. These programs (often called "indigent patient programs") are accessible through the Pharmaceutical Manufacturers' Association.

Medications included in this program range from contraceptives to chemotherapy. In fact, some manufacturers make available all their prescription products through their programs.

Eligibility requirements vary among the different manufacturers' programs. While some manufacturers have established very strict financial guidelines for participation, others leave the decision solely up to the patient's physician. For example, Marion Merrell Dow, Inc. allows the physician to determine patient need and in most cases, will provide a three-month supply of a product at a time. However, Marion Merrell Dow expects physicians to participate in this program by providing their services to these patients free of charge. While each of the programs varies according to its eligibility requirements, application

Over 50 pharmaceutical manufacturers offer free medication programs to people who wouldn't otherwise be able to afford medications.

to any of the programs must be made by a physician or through a hospital. All the companies require physicians to certify that the patient's diagnosis is correct for the drug therapy requested.

If you feel that you might be eligible for one of these programs, have your physician contact the Pharmaceuticals Manufacturers' Association at (800) PMA-INFO (762-4636) or in Washington, DC, call (202) 393-5200. When physicians provide the operator with the name of the prescription medicine they require, the operator will refer the physician to the appropriate company's program. We have also provided the numbers of individual drug company programs, which you may give to your physician. Note: These are not patient information lines. Only physicians are able to obtain information through them. So, give these numbers or addresses to your doctor, but, do not call them yourself.

Some of the companies currently participating in prescription drug indigent patient programs include:

Adria Laboratories—(800) 366-5570
Medications covered by program: various oncology products
Eligibility: Patients unable to afford the cost of the medication who have exhausted all Medicaid, Medicare, third-party insurance, and all resources from social agencies. The company requests that the physician provide his/her services for administering the drug at no charge.

Allergan, Inc.—(800) 347-4500
Medications covered by program: most products
Eligibility: Determined by physician, in the case of most products.

American Cyanamid Company, Lederle Laboratories Division—(800) 533-2273
Medications covered by program: all Lederle pharmaceutical products
Eligibility: Indigent patients ineligible for insurance or Medicaid.

Amgen Inc.—(800) 272-9376

Medications covered by program: Epogen; Neupogen

Eligibility: Low-income, uninsured, underinsured patients.

Ares-Serono, Inc.—(617) 982-9000

Medication covered by program: Metrodin

Eligibility: Patients without prescription medication insurance or patients who are not covered by public health programs.

Astra Pharmaceutical Products, Inc.—(800) 488-3247

Medications covered by program: Foscavir Injection

Eligibility: Patients without prescription medication insurance or patients who are not covered by public health programs.

Berlex Laboratories—(800) 473-7539

Medications covered by program: Fludara Injection

Eligibility: Patients not covered by Medicare, Medicaid, or private insurance with an annual income of less than $25,000 (for an individual patient) or $40,000 (for a patient with a family). Physician must provide his/her services free of charge to the patient.

Boehringer Ingelheim Pharmaceuticals, Inc.—(800) 556-8317

Medications covered by program: various products

Eligibility: Patients with financial hardship who are without prescription medication insurance or patients who are not covered by public health programs.

Boots Pharmaceuticals, Inc.

Boots Cares
Department CO
Boots Pharmaceuticals, Inc.
300 Tri-State International Office Center
Suite 200
Lincolnshire, IL 60069-4415
Product covered by program: Synthroid Tablets

Eligibility: Indigent patients.

Bristol-Meyers Squibb Company—(800) 736-0003

Products covered by program: various medications

Eligibility: Patients with financial hardship who are without prescription drug insurance or patients who are not covered by public health programs.

Burroughs Wellcome Company—(800) 722-9294

Products covered by program: all prescription medications

Eligibility: All other funding sources unavailable to patient with income below federal poverty guidelines.

Central Pharmaceuticals, Inc.—(301) 881-3052

Product covered by program: Niferex-150 Capsules

Eligibility: Limited to 5,000 patients; administered through the American Kidney Fund.

CIBA Pharmaceuticals—(800) 257-3273

Products covered by program: Most medications

Eligibility: Patients with financial hardship who are without prescription drug insurance or patients who are not covered by public health programs.

Connaught Laboratories, Inc.—
(717) 839-4617; (717) 839-7235 (fax)

Product covered by program: TheraCys

Eligibility: Patients with financial hardship who are uninsured and ineligible for Medicare and Medicaid.

DuPont Pharmaceuticals

Direct requests to local company sales representative.

Products covered by program: All non-controlled prescription medications

Eligibility: Patients with financial hardship who are ineligible for public assistance programs.

Fisons Pharmaceuticals

Fisons Respiratory Care Program
Fison Pharmaceuticals
P.O. Box 1766
Rochester, NY 14603
Products covered by program: Respiratory care products
Eligibility: Patients without private insurance or public assistance

and with annual household income of not more than $9000 for one or two people; allowance of $1000 per dependent child, with a total of up to $12,000 household income.

Genentech, Inc.—(800) 879-4747, ext. 1021

Products covered by program: Actimmune, Activase, Protropin

Eligibility: Uninsured patients who are unable to afford therapy and who are ineligible for any public assistance.

Glaxo, Inc.—(800) 452-9677

Products covered by program: All current medications

Eligibility: Indigent patients ineligible for public assistance programs or private insurance. Physician must waive his or her fee.

Hoechst-Roussel Pharmaceuticals, Inc.—(800) 422-4779

Product covered by program: Prokine

Eligibility: Patients with financial hardship, uninsured and ineligible for Medicaid.

Immunex Corporation—(206) 587-0430

Products covered by program: Leukine, Hydrea

Eligibility: Patients with financial hardship without private insurance and ineligible for public programs.

Janssen Pharmaceutical—(800) 544-2987

Product covered by program: Ergamisol

Eligibility: Patients with income less than $25,000 (total household) for whom purchase would cause hardship. Patient can have Medicare or insurance but no prescription coverage. Physician must waive his or her fee.

Knoll Pharmaceuticals—(800) 524-2474

Products covered by program: Isoptin, Rythmol, Santyl, Zostrix

Eligibility: Determined by the company based on physician request.

Eli Lilly and Company—(800) 545-5979

Products covered by program: Most prescription medications

Eligibility: Patients with limited resources and lacking third-party assistance.

Marion Merrell Dow, Inc.—(800) 362-7466

Products covered by program: All prescription medications

Eligibility: Indigent patients without insurance or other health care coverage. Physicians are encouraged to provide their services free of charge.

McNeil Pharmaceutical

Thomas Schwend, R.Ph.
Manager, Medical Information
McNeil Pharmaceutical
P.O. Box 300, Route 202 South
Raritan, NJ 08869-0602

Products covered by program: Various prescription medications

Eligibility: Indigent patients without prescription insurance coverage.

Merck Human Health Division—(800) 637-2579

Products covered by program: All except injectables

Eligibility: Patients with financial hardship who are without private insurance or who are ineligible for government assistance.

Miles Inc., Pharmaceutical Division—(203) 937-2000

Products covered by program: All

Eligibility: Patients with income below federal poverty level guidelines, who are not covered by private insurance and are ineligible for government-funded assistance programs.

Ortho Biotech—(800) 447-3437

Product covered by program: PROCRIT (epoetin alfa), for non-dialysis use

Eligibility: Available to any person who needs this medication and is without financial resources, including third-party insurance or government program assistance. Physicians are required to provide their services at no charge.

Parke-Davis, Division of Warner-Lambert Company—(800) 755-0120

Products covered by program: all pharmaceuticals

Eligibility: Patients of insufficient financial means and who have no medical plan coverage.

Pfizer Inc., Pfizer Labs Division, Roerig Division, Pratt Pharmaceuticals Division—(800) 646-4455

Products covered by program: All Pfizer outpatient products

Eligibility: Patients who are not eligible for third-party or Medicaid reimbursements for medications. Physicians are required to provide their services to the patient at no charge.

Pfizer Inc., Roerig Division—(800) 869-9979

Product covered by program: Diflucan

Eligibility: Patients without insurance, other third-party payers, Medicaid, and not eligible for the state's AIDS drug assistance program. Patient annual income must be below $25,000 (for individuals) and $40,000 (for families).

Pfizer Inc., Roerig Division, Pfizer Labs, Pratt Pharmaceuticals Division–The Arkansas Health Care Access Program—
(800) 950-8233; (501) 221-3033

Products covered by program: All Pfizer products

Eligibility: Individuals certified as eligible by the Arkansas Local County Department of Human Services. Physicians must waive all fees. This program is not applicable during hospital inpatient stays.

Pfizer, Roerig Division, Pfizer Labs, Pratt Pharmaceuticals Division–The Kentucky Health Care Access Program—
(606) 255-7442

Products covered by program: All Pfizer products

Eligibility: Individuals certified as eligible by the Kentucky Cabinet for Human Resources. Physicians must waive all fees. This program is not applicable during hospital inpatient stays.

Procter & Gamble Pharmaceuticals, Inc.—(800) 448-4878

Products covered by program: All P & G pharmaceutical products with a National Drug Code (NDC) beginning with 00149

Eligibility: Need and eligibility is determined by the physician.

Rhone-Poulenc Rorer Inc.—(215) 454-8298

Products covered by program: All

Eligibility: Need and eligibility is determined by the physician.

Roche Laboratories—(800) 526-6367, teleprompt #2
Products covered by program: full product line

Eligibility: Private practice outpatients who lack means to pay for their medications. Physicians make the determination.

Roxane Laboratories—(800) 274-8651
Product covered by program: Marinol Capsules

Eligibility: Available to uninsured patients with an annual income of less than $25,000 (without dependents) and less than $40,000 (with dependents).

Sandoz Pharmaceuticals Corporation—(800) 447-6673
Products covered by program: Clozaril; Eldepryl; Sandimmune; Sandoglobulin; Sandostatin; Parlodel

Eligibility: Trained staff make independent determination of patient need.

Sanofi Winthrop Pharmaceuticals—(800) 446-6267
Products covered by program: Selected medications

Eligibility: Contact local representative for details.

Schering Laboratories/Key Pharmaceuticals—(908) 298-4797 (fax)
Products covered by program: Intron A/Eulexin
All Other Products–Contact:
Schering Labs/Key Pharmaceuticals Drug Information Services—(908) 298-2188 (fax)

Eligibility: Patients who are truly in need and without resources, private or public, for their treatment. An internal assessment and a physician evaluation are required.

Searle—(800) 542-2526; (708) 470-6633 (fax)
Products covered by program: Aldactazide; Aldactone sustained releases; Kerlone; Calan; Nitrodisc; Norpace; Norpace CR extended-release; Cytotec; Maxiquin.

Eligibility: The physician is the sole determinant of a patient's eligibility.

SmithKline Beecham Pharmaceuticals Compassionate Care Programs—(800) 866-6273; (202) 637-6695

Products covered by program: Eminase; Triostat

Eligibility: Patients must be without private or public insurance and have an annual income of less than $18,000 (single) or $25,000 (family).

SmithKline Beecham Pharmaceuticals Access to Care Program—(215) 751-5722; (800) 546-0420

Products covered by program: Tagamet; Augmentin; Relafen; Dyazide; Compazine; Bectroban; Amoxil; Ridaura; all other SKB products

Eligibility: Completely determined by physician.

Syntex Laboratories—(800) 444-4200 Cytovene Medical Information Line; (800) 822-8255 Physician's Request Line

Product covered by program: Cytovene

Eligibility: Patients without means to purchase the medication and not eligible for any form of third-party reimbursement.

3M Pharmaceuticals—(800) 328-0255

Products covered by program: Most drug products

Eligibility: Patients with financial hardship who are not covered by insurance or public assistance programs.

The Upjohn Company—(616) 329-8244

Products covered by program: All

Eligibility: Patients with financial hardship who are not covered by insurance or public assistance programs.

Wyeth-Ayerst Laboratories–Norplant Foundation—(703) 706-5933

Products covered by program: Norplant

Eligibility: Patients with financial hardship who are not covered by insurance or public assistance programs.

Wyeth-Ayerst Laboratories

Roger J. Eurbin
Professional Services IPP
555 E. Lancaster Avenue
St. Davids, PA 19087

Products covered by program: Various

Eligibility: Indigent patients who are not covered by insurance or public assistance programs.

HOW TO SAVE MONEY ON HOSPITAL BILLS

Where do Americans spend most of their health care dollars? At doctors' offices or at hospitals?

It's not even a contest. As expensive as doctors' bills may be, twice as much money is spent on hospital care each year. In 1990, hospital services accounted for 38 percent of the $666.2 billion spent on health care in the United States, compared to 23 percent for personal health care services (such as drugs, medical equipment and dentistry) and 19 percent for physicians' services.

The message: Hospital care doesn't come cheap. And, at the same time you're watching the hospital bills pile up, you may be asking yourself, "Do I really even need to be hospitalized at all?" In this chapter, we'll show you how to get answers to that question and save money in the process.

Is Hospitalization Always Really Necessary?

The most obvious way to save money on hospital bills is to avoid hospitalization completely whenever possible. Thousands of hospital admissions and procedures are absolutely inappropriate. Yes, as surprising as it might seem, people are sometimes admitted to the hospital unnecessarily. But even when hospitalization is essential, a hospital stay may become significantly longer—and more costly— than necessary.

Just consider the startling findings of a study published in the *New England Journal of Medicine* in 1986. It suggested that as many as 40 percent of hospitalizations of nonelderly patients could be avoided. Researchers reviewed the medical records of more than 1,100 hospi-

> The most obvious way to save
> money on hospital bills is to
> avoid hospitalization com-
> pletely whenever possible.

talized patients, and concluded not only that 23 percent of hospitalizations were completely unnecessary, but also that an additional 17 percent of hospital admissions could have been averted by using ambulatory or outpatient surgery.

Other research has reached similar conclusions. A 1991 study found that 54 percent of all hospital days spent on medical wards were unjustified. So was 40 percent of the time spent on surgical wards and 26 percent of the time on pediatric wards. That's a lot of wasted time and money, not to mention the stress and strain on patients and their families.

HOW DO UNNECESSARY HOSPITALIZATIONS HAPPEN?

In these cost-conscious times, why is so much extra time being spent in the hospital? After all, aren't doctors becoming more careful than ever about reserving hospitalization only for patients who are extremely sick, and then discharging them as soon as they're well enough to go home? Well, that's the way it should be. But unnecessary hospitalizations and overly long hospital stays still occur. Consider the following common scenarios:

- You are admitted to a hospital for an acute illness, even though you could be treated as an outpatient, even in a doctor's office.

- You enter a hospital for surgery that could have been done on an outpatient basis.

- You are hospitalized in order to undergo diagnostic proce-dures, which could have been conducted outside the hospital.

- You are admitted to a hospital when your situation really called for a different type of setting that may have been unavailable—perhaps nursing or home health care.

Nowadays, there are strong pressures from the government and insurance companies to minimize hospital admissions, and to dis-charge patients earlier than in previous years. Although these efforts are seen primarily as a cost-saving measure, they are also often good medicine. In fact, if you are hospitalized and your stay drags on and on, there's a good chance that your hospital stay is lengthier than it needs to be from a medical standpoint—not to mention that it's unnecessarily expensive.

Questions to Ask Your Doctor

"That infection just isn't getting any better. In fact, it seems to be getting worse. I think it's time for you to go to the hospital."

Thousands of times each day across the country, doctors are making recommendations like this to their patients, often providing little or no more information on why a hospital stay is essential. That's not good enough. If you ever find yourself in this situation, don't just nod your head in agreement. Become a more active patient and do some investigative work of your own to ensure that there's no alternative other than hospitalization. No matter what the reason for your impending stay in the hospital, following are some questions you need to ask (although the questions may vary depending on your medical condition and whether you're entering the hospital for surgery or for some other reason).

DOCTOR, WHY DO I NEED
TO BE ADMITTED TO THE HOSPITAL?

If you're so ill that your doctor feels that hospitalization is required, you probably already know what's wrong with you. But if there's anything you don't understand, get your questions answered. Don't settle for brief or incomplete information from your doctor. If his or her explanation is, "You've got a kidney infection," or "You've got problems with your lungs," demand a more thorough answer. Ask for the precise medical terminology that describes your condition and, if necessary, write it down to make sure you'll remember it. These technical words sometimes sound like a foreign language, but it's important for you to know them, particularly if you decide to consult another physician for a second opinion.

Make sure your doctor also explains what risks are associated with your illness if you do *not* enter the hospital—as well as the risks of the treatment and procedures planned for you in the hospital. Ask what the chances are that your therapy will be successful and what alternative treatments are available.

CAN I BE TREATED FOR MY ILLNESS AS AN OUTPATIENT?

Many medical conditions do not require hospitalization, particularly if you agree to work closely with your doctor in an outpatient setting. Let your physician know that if you can be treated outside the hospital, you're willing to make frequent office visits so your response to therapy and your overall progress can be monitored.

Of course, doctors' visits themselves aren't inexpensive. But they will still be considerably less than the enormous charges associated with hospitalization. And, remember, if you're admitted to the hospital, you'll still have to pay a fee for your physician's hospital visits.

At first glance, it might seem unrealistic to think that you could actually receive adequate care at home for something your doctor had initially advised hospitalization. But that's sometimes the case. In certain situations, home care can provide you with quality medical services administered by trained health care professionals while you're surrounded by all the comforts of home. For instance, let's say that you need a course of intravenous (IV) antibiotics. It may not be necessary to enter the hospital to receive it, since a qualified nurse could come to your house to administer it. Or ask your doctor if oral antibiotics (taken by mouth) might be tried first before he or she prescribes IV medications; if the oral therapy fails, then you could consider the IV treatment, at home or in the hospital.

"WHY DO I NEED SURGERY?"

If your doctor has recommended admission to the hospital because you need to have an operation, make sure you fully understand the procedure and why it needs to be performed. Keep in mind an obvious fact: It's your body. Thus, you have the right to know everything that's going to happen to you. As you talk to your doctor, ask whether the operation could be postponed, and whether the surgery might be less successful if you wait.

Some doctors would be quite content if you didn't ask any questions at all. But don't be intimidated if your own doctor seems to brush off your questions with only brief, indifferent answers and an impatient look. If the doctor's full explanation is, "You have a hernia," for instance, you're entitled to more information. Okay, so you have a hernia—but what if it had never even bothered you, and you hadn't even known that you had a hernia until now? Is it really essential that the hernia be surgically repaired? Bear in mind that no surgery is risk-free and, with most procedures, there are potential complications. So be sure to inquire about the risks of an operation, and what complications could occur. Ask your doctor to discuss the pros and cons of the surgery with you.

> *There is no such thing as minor surgery. For that reason,* never *take surgery lightly.*

ARE THERE ALTERNATIVES TO HAVING SURGERY?

There is no such thing as minor surgery. For that reason, *never* take surgery lightly. In most cases, it should be considered a last-resort procedure. Not only is surgery expensive, but it also tends to carry greater risks than more conservative therapy. Always ask your doctor what your other options are. Is there a more conservative, less invasive approach that could be tried instead of surgery? For example: If your doctor advises a diskectomy to ease back pain associated with a herniated disk, ask if it can be treated in other ways, such as with bed rest or exercise.

Of course, there are times when surgery is the right choice. Maybe you've already tried alternative procedures with no success. Or perhaps they just aren't appropriate. When your doctor recommends coronary artery bypass surgery, for instance, his or her decision may be based on the severity of blockages in your coronary arteries, and which of those arteries are most seriously affected. You may be at risk for a heart attack if surgery isn't done immediately. However, doctors can differ about the best approach to take. If you're not satisfied with your doctor's explanation, talk to a second or a third doctor until you *are* satisfied.

CAN THE SURGERY BE DONE ON AN OUTPATIENT BASIS?

A growing number of operations do not require admission to a hospital. Whether you're having a hernia repair or cataract surgery, you may be a good candidate for having the procedure done at an ambulatory surgery center, which might even be affiliated with the hospital to which you otherwise would have been admitted. We'll discuss this option in detail later in the chapter.

Choose a Hospital Carefully

Let's say that you've agreed with your doctor (and with the physician providing a second opinion) that you need to be hospitalized, whether for medical treatment or for surgery. Your next decision is a critical one: To what hospital should you be admitted? There may be a half-dozen or more hospitals in your city, and your selection of the right facility could literally be a matter of life or death!

In the past, you may not have played a part in this decision. In fact, most patients still don't. They simply go to the hospital that their doctor recommends. Your own physician has probably been granted "privileges" at one or more hospitals, meaning that the medical board at those facilities awarded the doctor the privilege of admitting patients. But more needs to go into your decision than your doctor's affiliations. You need to choose a hospital that has a good track record in caring for your particular medical condition.

Keep this important fact in mind: All hospitals are not the same. Their fees can vary considerably, although money isn't the only thing you should be thinking about. You need to look for *quality,* too. There are many excellent hospitals—and probably just as many poor ones—and while it's common to equate price with quality, this does not apply to health care. In fact, you will probably find that some of the best hospitals may cost the least, while some of the worst are among the most expensive.

DO YOUR HOMEWORK

Don't hesitate to call hospitals in your community and ask for quotes on their room charges, their operating room fees, and other expenses. However, these fees can be deceiving. Some hospitals actually *undercharge* for room and board, and use this pricing strategy as a means of attracting patients. Later, when the hospital bill is finally presented, the patient is usually shocked to find that the bill includes dozens of separate charges for items such as a bar of soap or a bottle of shampoo. Welcome to the sneaky world of hospital fees!

> *Don't hesitate to call hospitals in your community and ask for quotes on their room charges, their operating room fees, and other expenses.*

As you're calling around, ask hospital administrators about ways in which the hospital bill can be reduced. For example, some hospitals offer discounts if you pay your bill upfront, rather than waiting for payment by the insurance company. Ultimately, of course, you'd be reimbursed by your insurance company, while saving some money in the process. Thus, if you can afford it—and admittedly, many people can't—you can reduce your total bill by paying for charges in advance, which means reducing your own co-payment, too.

HOW TO ASSESS A HOSPITAL'S QUALITY

While you're evaluating hospital fees, spend just as much (or more) time assessing quality, too. Frankly, a low-cost hospital isn't worth much if it provides poor quality care.

At any given time, at any given hospital, you may receive either excellent or awful treatment. But just as some brokerage houses or banks generally provide better overall returns on investments than others, patients generally fare better in some hospitals than they do in others. Before ever entering a particular hospital as a patient, you need to find out everything you can about its quality of care—from its malpractice history to its patient death rates.

Where can you turn for this kind of information? Here are a few ideas:

TALK TO YOUR DOCTOR   Your physician is probably familiar with most hospitals in your community, and he or she may have privileges at several of them. Ask your doctor for help in evaluating which hospital would be best for your specific needs (i.e., is there one that has more experience in performing the type of surgery you need?).

INQUIRE AT THE HOSPITALS THEMSELVES   Call several hospitals and ask about their track record in caring for patients, particularly for the condition for which you're being hospitalized. Hospitals keep track of how patients fare in their wards. They know the average length of hospital stays. They know the frequency with which unexpected compli-

Is the Hospital Accredited?

When you're looking into the quality of a particular hospital, be sure to find out its accreditation status. Every three years, hospitals are visited by inspectors from a government-sanctioned organization—the Joint Commission on Accreditation of Healthcare Organizations (JCAHO)—that can award accreditation to hospitals. The investigators, usually doctors and nurses, determine whether hospitals meet established guidelines for quality of care and services, evaluating criteria such as procedures in intensive care units, nursing care, medical recordkeeping, and the safety of equipment such as x-ray machines.

JCAHO can award full accreditation to a hospital or it may give conditional accreditation instead to a hospital that is not up to standard, while establishing a time period by which shortcomings must be corrected in order for full accreditation to be granted. And while accreditation is a voluntary process, most hospitals consider it extremely important. Without accreditation, hospitals cannot receive Medicare payments from the federal government for the care of elderly patients.

So is hospital accreditation a guarantee that you'll receive excellent care? The simple answer is "no." Even so, it is an indication that the facility has at least met the government's minimum standards. For that reason, it may mean more in terms of quality than a mere license, which every hospital must have.

To find out if a particular hospital is accredited, you can contact JCAHO directly at (202) 434-4525. However, while letting you know whether a hospital is accredited, JCAHO will not necessarily reveal why a particular hospital was denied full accreditation. In a few states, these accreditation reports may be made public, although they remain confidential in most parts of the country.

cations occur. They know the rates of patient deaths. These statistics are good gauges of the quality of care that a hospital provides. In California, for example, the mortality for Medicare patients undergoing surgical gallbladder removals (cholecystectomies) ranges from nearly zero to 19 percent. Thus, at the hospital at the worst end of the scale, your chances of dying when your gallbladder is removed are nearly one in five, 19 times higher than at some other hospitals. If you're looking for peace of mind, you'd certainly feel more secure as a patient in a hospital where the mortality rate is low.

> *Before ever entering a particular hospital as a patient, you need to find out everything you can about its quality of care—from its malpractice history to its patient death rates.*

CHECK OUT GOVERNMENT AND OTHER STATISTICS Hospitals aren't the only ones keeping records on their performance. Government agencies and private watchdog groups also analyze "patient outcomes" at hospitals throughout the country. A close look at the results can be quite revealing. Some hospitals are good or bad in specialized areas. Others are good or bad across the board, no matter what condition is being treated. If a hospital has a low cesarean section rate, for instance, it probably has close controls and peer review over the way its doctors practice medicine; on the other hand, a high cesarean rate may indicate that doctors have too much freedom in deciding when to perform this operation.

A study published in 1989 confirmed what many doctors and patients had long suspected: The more experience doctors and staff have with a particular surgery, the more likely they are to perform it well. The study found that in hospitals where high numbers of certain surgical procedures are performed, there tend to be significantly fewer deaths associated with those operations. Yet as useful as this information can be, we don't believe that it has been as accessible to consumers as it should be—but that's changing. Various organizations are gaining access to this information, and are making it available to the public at large.

One of the best resources we've seen is *Consumers' Guide to Hospitals*, published by the Center for the Study of Services. It presents death

Choosing Hospitals: How Do They Compare?

Your choice of a hospital could determine just how well you'll fare in its operating room and on its medical wards. In the *Consumers' Guide to Hospitals*, based on data from the government's Health Care Financing Administration, you can find death rate statistics for thousands of hospitals, including analyses of patient outcomes for conditions like gallbladder removal, acute myocardial infarction (heart attack), pneumonia/influenza, stroke, hip fracture, and initial pacemaker insertion. In an attempt to be fair, the book adjusts these figures to compensate for the fact that some hospitals tend to see sicker or more frail patients than others.

To see just how eye-opening and useful these statistics can be, let's look at some examples drawn from the 1992 edition of the *Consumers' Guide to Hospitals:*

If you live in the city of St. Louis, Missouri, and need to have a pacemaker inserted, you could choose from among many hospitals. Here is just a sampling of them, along with their mortality rates when a pacemaker is initially implanted.

	Cases	Adjusted Death Rate
St. Louis University Medical Center	79	0.0%
Deaconess Hospital	86	1.0%
St. Anthony's Medical Center	90	4.7%
Bethesda General Hospital	15	6.9%
Central Medical Center	7	24.5%

Which hospital would you pick? You could use the information provided above to make an educated decision based on (1) which hospitals have the most experience in pacemaker insertion and (2) which have the lowest death rates.

Below are figures for gallbladder removal in a sampling of hospitals in Houston. Again, you could use this information as a basis for discussion with your doctor when you're trying to decide which facility is best for you:

	Cases	Adjusted Death Rate
AMI Heights Hospital	93	0.0%
Hermann Hospital	89	0.9%
Houston Northwest Medical Center	19	2.1%
Rosewood Medical Center	20	6.4%
Doctors Hospital East Loop	14	14.8%

rates by condition at nearly 6,000 hospitals in the U.S., using data on Medicare patients collected by the federal government. It also provides background information about the hospitals themselves, such as how many of their physicians are board-certified, and which hospitals have advanced training programs for physicians.

For a look at how hospitals and medical centers differ in patient outcomes, see the box opposite.

Cutting Your Hospital Costs

Although hospital care is extremely expensive, there are strategies that can help you reduce your hospital bill. One of the best overall approaches is simple: Spend as little time in the hospital as possible. And that means learning the hospital's rules in order to play the game. Here are some common ones:

Know When to Check In and Out

Hospitals aren't exactly hotels. Even so, there are some parallels between them, such as daily room charges (which include housekeeping) and even check-in and check-out times. As with a hotel, if you arrive at the hospital early or leave late, you will be charged for an extra day.

If you're being admitted for an elective procedure, call ahead and ask the hospital about check-in time, and then abide by it. When you're ready to be discharged, be prompt about going home on time to avoid extra fees. Even if the friend or relative who is driving you home can't arrive until later in the day, check out before he or she gets there. Most hospitals have sitting rooms where you can wait for your transportation and not worry about being exposed to additional charges.

AVOID HOSPITAL "DOWN TIMES"

Although hospital administrators will tell you that their facilities provide "round-the-clock services," the care at various times of the day can vary dramatically. Hospitals do not function the same at 2:00 in the morning as they do at 2:00 in the afternoon, nor are their services the same on a Sunday as they are on a weekday.

Yes, there are nurses and other personnel on duty 24 hours a day. But nights, weekends and holidays are generally difficult times to get things done in a hospital. Laboratories close down or operate with a reduced staff. Tests may be delayed until the following day, even if it means postponing your discharge to get them done. Doctors may have weekends off, and their approval of a particular procedure or decision will be held up until their return. So while you might be ready to go home on a Sunday morning, the covering physician may decide to keep you until your own doctor returns on Monday. And all the while, your hospital expenses will be accumulating.

In a revealing study published in *Medical Care* in 1989, researchers examined the medically unnecessary hospital delays that occurred in one medical center in New England. They found that a full 30 percent of all hospitalized patients experienced an unnecessary delay that postponed their discharge and thus increased their hospital bill. These delays, which resulted in an average of 2.9 days of additional hospitalization, were caused by such things as poor scheduling of tests, slow physician decision-making, and faulty discharge planning. These delays were responsible for 17 percent of all days spent in the hospital.

If you need to undergo nonemergency surgery, keep in mind that many hospitals have very busy surgical calendars, which can delay your operation for days. Have your doctor schedule your surgery as much in advance as possible. Also, don't expect an elective procedure to be performed on weekends; instead, it will probably be delayed until the following week. If you get caught in a hospital on a weekend, you may find yourself waiting for your surgery.

DEMAND TIMELY TESTING

At times, the only thing standing between you and discharge from the hospital is a test or two. But in a busy medical center, it can actually be days before that test is scheduled. Some hospitals have a policy in which tests aren't conducted at all after 5 p.m., or at any time on the weekend. So if your doctor orders a test on Friday afternoon, you may have to wait until Monday or even later for it to be performed.

Imagine how frustrating—and costly—this situation can be. However, you may have other options. For instance, ask your doctor if the test can be done on an outpatient basis. Depending on the particular test and the reason it has been ordered, you might be able to go home and then return later—either to the hospital or to your doctor's office—to have the test.

Even if the test itself needs to be performed while you're hospitalized, ask if you can go home before the results arrive on your doctor's desk. Some test reports take days to come back, and if you're waiting for them while in the hospital, it can be a costly wait indeed.

Don't Go to the Hospital Empty-Handed

Here's a universal axiom about hospital life: Nothing is free. Everything costs money—and generally a lot more money than it costs outside the hospital walls. Most items have an astronomical markup, and since hospitals have a captive audience in patients, the exorbitant bills are generally paid without much complaint.

For example, would you believe that two aspirin could cost $7 in the hospital? That's exactly what we discovered in a recent conversation with a pharmacist at a large medical center in Los Angeles. Hospitals charge a minimum fee for every pill they dispense, even if it's a simple and inexpensive medication like aspirin, so expect your wallet to be gouged.

You can fight back, however, winning some of the small battles even if you don't win the war. Here are two suggestions:

- Bring basic toiletry items such as shampoo with you to the hospital. If you obtained them from the hospital instead, they would show up on your hospital bill—and in a big way. When one of us was recently hospitalized, our bill ended up showing a $14 charge for a disposable razor! Any way you look at it, that's an expensive shave.

- All new medications that your doctor prescribes during your hospitalization—such as antibiotics for pneumonia, or steroids for an acute asthma attack—are best ordered through the hospital's own pharmacy. But if you have already been taking other medications outside the hospital, perhaps a cholesterol-lowering drug or postmenopausal estrogen replacement, ask your doctor about bringing your own supply with you to the hospital—thus avoiding the hospital's markups.

Explain to your doctor that you didn't realize that hospitalization required taking a vow of poverty. Ask for a discharge as soon as possible, promising to return to your doctor's office when the test results arrive, particularly if any changes in your treatment need to be made.

Sometimes, your physician will say, "Sorry, but I need to see these test results before I'd feel comfortable discharging you." If that means waiting a few extra days for that test to be conducted and the results to reach your doctor's desk, try to do some negotiating to reduce your fees. Contact the hospital's business office, and explain matter of factly the reasons why you're not being discharged: namely, because the hospital is unable to schedule the test and deliver its results in a timely manner. Tell them that since the hospital is responsible for this delay, it should bear a portion of the costs of your extended stay. Be assertive. You might save some money in the process.

One other important point: To cut down on your health care costs, ask your doctor about taking certain tests *before* you are admitted to the hospital. In general, routine tests will be much less expensive if they're conducted on an outpatient basis, particularly since you'll be able to avoid a day or two of hospitalization. And if the tests turn up a problem that would delay your surgery, you will have detected it *before* you begin running up enormous hospital bills.

LIMIT DELAYS IN CONSULTATIONS

If your condition is particularly complicated, your own doctor may ask another physician (usually a specialist in a relevant field) to review your case and provide advice on the course of your treatment. For example, let's say that your internist is treating you for pneumonia. After two days in the hospital, you suddenly develop a severe and unusual rash. Your internist may ask a dermatologist (a doctor specializing in the treatment of skin disorders) to become involved in your care, examining the rash and recommending ways to treat it.

At times, however, this consultation process can be painfully slow. If your case is not considered an emergency, days may pass before the consultant can examine you and then discuss his or her findings with your own doctor. If your physician insists that the consultant's input is essential before you can go home, you could be stuck in your hospital room, playing solitaire or watching television.

As much as you'd like your doctor to be your strongest advocate in this situation, don't count on it. Your doctor may have a dozen or more other hospitalized patients to tend to, plus a full schedule of patients to see in the office, and resolving delays in the consultation process may be low on the priority list. That means you're going to have

> *Ask your doctor about taking certain tests before you are admitted to the hospital.*

to take the initiative. Insist on discussing the problem with your doctor. Or even pick up the phone and call the consultant's office yourself. Explain that his or her timely care is the only thing standing between you and the comfort of your own home. If you don't get results, ask your doctor to find a different consultant.

MINIMIZE OTHER DELAYS

In what other ways can you combat delays and red tape? If you have a choice in the matter, we suggest entering a hospital at the beginning of the week. Particularly if your stay is short, you'll be out before the weekend when activity slows down in the hospital. In the same way, avoid having elective surgery the day before a major holiday such as Thanksgiving. Chances are your postoperative care will suffer, and by the time you get home, the Thanksgiving turkey will be dry.

Also, since it is ultimately your physician who will decide when you will go home, continue to keep the communication channels open. If you're not careful, you can easily become quite isolated from your doctor. So, rather than allowing your doctor to make decisions in a vacuum without any input from you, request a full explanation of his or her actions. Why is a test being scheduled for tomorrow rather than today? Why are you being discharged on Thursday instead of Wednesday? Can the discharge orders be written early in the day so there is time for the hospital staff to prepare for your departure before the day is over?

By becoming an active participant in this process, you may force your doctor to reevaluate the way hospitalized patients are cared for, rather than making decisions by rote. Along the way, you're more likely to keep wasted days in the hospital to a minimum. One study concluded that when doctors kept daily logs in which they had to explain and support each day their patients were hospitalized, the number of patients subjected to unnecessary days in the hospital dipped by about ten percent.

Don't forget that a competent, understanding doctor can become your best ally in the hospital. He or she understands how hospitals work, and can help ensure that you don't get lost in the bureaucratic shuffle. If you need to see specialists, your doctor can help ensure that this is done promptly. And if you're unhappy with your care, your doctor can add leverage to your complaints.

Is "Same Day Surgery" For You?

If your surgery is scheduled for Tuesday, how important is it for you to arrive at the hospital on Monday? Depending on the operation, some doctors believe an early arrival isn't necessary at all. That may even be the case for major surgery.

Gaining in popularity is "same day surgery," in which hospital check-in is on the day of the operation, not before. It's convenient—and it instantly cuts a day off the cost of hospitalization.

Some people find other advantages to same day surgery. They dread the day (and night) before surgery, when worry and anxiety levels can become absolutely overwhelming. If you can stay at home, however, keeping occupied and spending time with family and friends in familiar surroundings, you'll probably reduce your fear of surgery. Many people report that they slept very poorly in the hospital on the night before their operation. At home, however, they're more likely to get a better night's sleep.

Talk with your surgeon about the possibility of same day admission. Particularly as doctors and hospitals increase efforts to keep hospital costs under control, your own doctor may be agreeable to the idea, unless you have a medical problem (such as diabetes) that needs special attention before the surgery, or if particular procedures need to be performed the night before your operation.

DON'T CAUSE DELAYS YOURSELF

When assigning blame for extended hospitalizations, don't overlook your own role in this process. Patients are often asked to make tough decisions about their care, such as giving approval for a particular procedure that may carry some risks. Understandably, it's hard to make these decisions instantaneously. At the same time, you need to keep in mind that while you're hospitalized, charges for your care are continuing around the clock. It's to your advantage to talk with your doctor and family members and make important decisions without unusual delays.

AVOID BREAKDOWNS IN DISCHARGE PLANNING

Sometimes, you may have your bags packed, ready to leave the hospital. But if your doctor's discharge orders have assigned you to go to a nursing home or rehabilitation center rather than back to your own home—and space isn't available in that facility—you may be relegated to a state of limbo, marooned in the hospital with no way out. Patients can wait weeks or even months for a space in the most sought-after facilities.

What's the answer? If your doctor has told you that you may need placement in a nursing home or rehabilitation center after your hospitalization, begin making plans early. Most hospitals have social workers who can search for the appropriate facility, and make arrangements for your transfer to this facility as soon as space becomes available.

Look Over Your Hospital Bill Carefully

At the time of discharge, particularly from an inpatient hospitalization, you'll understandably be eager to go home. But first take a few minutes to review your hospital bill. Mistakes not only happen, they happen a lot. A study conducted by the federal government's General Accounting Office discovered that a startling 95 percent of all hospital bills contain errors! As you might suspect, most of these mistakes are in the hospital's favor, not·yours, with overcharges more the rule than the exception.

Most people take one look at their hospital bill, and don't know where to begin. First of all, the total at the bottom of the bill may take their breath away, and they may be too upset to wade their way through the fine print. Some of the bill may also be difficult to interpret. Many patients simply throw up their hands and say, "My insurance company will have to figure it all out!" After all, isn't the insurance company paying the bill anyway? Don't forget that your insurer is probably paying for only *part* of the bill. You are responsible for deductibles, co-payments, and any services that aren't covered in your policy. So by catching errors yourself, you will probably save some money.

ASK FOR AN ITEMIZED BILL

If you haven't been give an itemized bill, ask for one. It might look intimidating—it can be several pages long—but it should break down all your expenses, including charges for room and board, for each laboratory test, for every drug or medication, and for all medical supplies (heating pad, bedpan, thermometer, etc.). Don't accept bulk billings from labs, which might just lump all your lab charges into one charge. And ask for an explanation of anything marked "miscellaneous fees."

As you study the hospital bill, look to see if you were charged for anything twice. Or if you were charged for services you never received. Were you billed for a private room when you stayed in a semiprivate one? Were you charged for eight days, even though your hospital stay only lasted six days? Were you billed for a pint of blood for which there should not have been any charge, since a family member donated blood to replace the pint you used?

Sometimes the errors are obvious, like when an elderly woman is charged for a pregnancy test or a man is billed for a hysterectomy. But the mistakes are usually more subtle, and will require looking over the bill carefully and asking questions.

If the billing office or the hospital ombudsman (a staff member available to answer patient inquiries and resolve problems) won't answer all your questions, make it clear that you are ready to pay your bill as soon as you find out what you're being billed for—and not before! Emphasize that while you're willing to pay for services you received, you won't pay for those you didn't!

KEEP A HOSPITAL DIARY

What's the best way to keep a hospital honest? Some patients keep a diary of their hospital stay, and compare it with the hospital bill when it arrives. The diary is a record of your entire hospital-ization, listing every service that was provided and everything that happened. Here is some information that should be included:

> *A study conducted by the federal government's General Accounting Office discovered that a startling 95 percent of all hospital bills contain errors!*

WHAT PHYSICIANS DID YOU SEE EACH DAY?   Don't let your doctor charge you if he or she didn't see you on a particular day. Also, make a note of the amount of time the doctor spent with you; if he pops his head in and then is gone in the blink of an eye, you shouldn't be fully charged for an inpatient visit.

WHAT DID YOUR PHYSICIANS TELL YOU EACH DAY?   This information will help you figure out why you are hospitalized and what needs to happen before you will be discharged. It will also come in handy as you describe your progress to family members.

WHAT TESTS OR PROCEDURES WERE PERFORMED EACH DAY?   Ask your doctor to tell you the name of every test being ordered. Double-check the test by asking the technician who comes to draw your blood or who takes an x-ray to confirm what test you're having.

WHAT MEDICATIONS DID YOU RECEIVE EACH DAY?   Ask your nurse to identify each pill you are given, and how frequently you're supposed to take it. By writing down this information, you'll have a better chance of catching errors—either medications given too often or not often enough, or errors in the medication charges on your hospital bill.

When You're Told You Need Surgery

Hospitalization and surgery are expensive. Operations also require recuperation time. Thus, as you enter the hospital, you need to feel comfortable that you aren't becoming one of the many thousands of patients each year who endure unnecessary hospitalizations and surg-

What's the best way to keep a hospital honest? Some patients keep a diary of their hospital stay, and compare it with the hospital bill when it arrives.

eries. Yes, your doctor may make his or her best recommendation based on training and experience. But, to repeat, it's your body. The final decision is yours.

Be particularly cautious if your doctor recommends one of the following operations, which many studies have categorized as highly discretionary and often unnecessary:

- Tonsillectomy
- Cesarean section
- Hysterectomy
- Oophorectomy (removal of the ovaries)
- Hemorrhoidectomy
- Dilation and curettage (scraping of the uterine lining)
- Prostatectomy (removal of the prostate gland)
- Back surgery
- Hip/knee replacements
- Gallbladder surgery (cholecystectomy)
- Varicose vein removal
- Coronary artery bypass surgery
- Carotid endarterectomy (removal of plaque from a neck artery)

What do all of these procedures have in common? There is an element of subjectivity involved in each of them. If you were to fill a room with doctors and ask them to tell you whether the above procedures were necessary in particular cases, you'd probably hear a lot of disagreement. We strongly believe that these operations (and others) are performed much too often.

So what should you do if your own doctor recommends one of these procedures? Here's our advice: Take a step back and think carefully before you decide to go ahead with surgery. There might be more conservative approaches that can be used to treat your condition just as successfully. And *always* get a second opinion.

A 1986 study in the *New England Journal of Medicine* suggests that when a doctor makes a decision about surgery for a patient, it may be influenced by how widely the same procedure is used in his or her community. In fact, when researchers looked at the frequency with which certain operations were performed, they found wide variations from one part of the country to another. Coronary artery bypass surgery, for instance, occurred 3.1 times more often in some areas than in others. Carotid endarterectomy (an operation to increase blood flow in the arteries that carry blood to the brain) was used four times more frequently, and total hip replacement three times more often, in certain sections of the country than in others. For some procedures, the variation in use between sites was as much as 26 fold!

Let's briefly examine a number of other studies that have looked specifically at the frequency with which common surgeries or medical procedures are used inappropriately, and whether there are differences in their use in different medical settings:

- In a study published in 1993, researchers examined the use of three common procedures—coronary artery bypass surgery, coronary angiography, and balloon angioplasty—in the state of New York. They concluded that bypass surgery was used appropriately 91 percent of the time, compared to inappropriate use in 2 percent of cases, and uncertain appropriateness in the remaining 7 percent. The other procedures did not fare as well: Angiography and angioplasty were used appropriately in 76 percent and 58 percent of cases, respectively, and inappropriately in 4 percent of cases in each instance.

- A 1993 study from the Rand Corporation evaluated the appropriateness of hysterectomies in patients in seven health plans. The researchers found that, overall, about 16 percent of women underwent hysterectomies that were considered "clinically inappropriate." One of the health plans had a much higher rate of inappropriate hysterectomies—27 percent. The investigators concluded that "the inappropriate provision of surgical and medical procedures occurs throughout the health care delivery system."

- An earlier Rand Corporation study, published in 1987, looked at the use of three common procedures—coronary angiography, carotid endarterectomy, and endoscopy of the upper gastrointestinal (G.I.) tract. The researchers concluded that angiography was conducted appropriately 74 percent of the time, for equivocal reasons 9 percent of the time, and unnecessarily in 17 percent of cases. Carotid endarterectomy was used appropriately much less often (in 35 percent of cases), compared to 32 percent of cases categorized as equivocal, and 32 percent as unnecessary. Upper G.I. endoscopy was performed appropriately 72 percent of the time, inappropriately in 17 percent of cases, while its use in the remaining 11 percent was considered equivocal.

- A study published in *Medical Care* showed variations in the frequency of surgeries in a traditional fee-for-service setting, compared to a prepaid practice. The researchers found that procedures such as hysterectomies, tonsillectomies, appendectomies, and cholecystectomies (gallbladder removal) were performed nearly four times more often in fee-for-service medicine.

What's the message from all of these studies? Before you agree to any surgery, do your homework: Read as much as you can about the procedure; ask questions about alternatives; and get a second opinion. The operation you save could be your own.

WHAT ABOUT CESAREAN SECTIONS?

The utilization of cesarean sections (also called C-sections) to deliver babies has been studied extensively, and the findings are both revealing and disturbing. C-sections are not only the most common major surgical procedure in the U.S., but they are also the operation most often performed unnecessarily. Although C-sections pose an increased risk of complications and even death to the mother, nearly one of every four pregnant women nationwide can expect to have her baby delivered this way.

A 1992 report by Public Citizen's Health Research Group put it bluntly, stating that "the majority of American physicians, hospitals and insurers have continued sticking their heads in the sand and ignoring over a decade of evidence undeniably showing that American women are undergoing an onslaught of this unnecessary and dangerous surgery."

The Health Research Group's report found vast discrepancies in the C-section rates in various parts of the country, and from one hospital to another. For example, while Nevada had a C-section rate of 31.7 percent in 1989, Alaska's rate was only 15.2 percent. In some hospitals, C-sections accounted for *more than half* of all births—such as Abrom Kaplan Memorial Hospital in Louisiana (57.5 percent), Humboldt Hospital in Nevada (56.6 percent), and Williamson Appalachian Regional Hospital in Kentucky (55.4 percent).

> *If your doctor has recommended a nonemergency operation, always seek a second opinion.*

GET A SECOND OPINION

Our advice is simple: Take back control. If your doctor has recommended a nonemergency operation, always seek a second opinion. Your physician should not object to this decision—he or she might even be able to refer you to another doctor for another point of view—and, in fact, your insurance company may require it for certain procedures. Two doctors can look at the same diagnosis, the same x-rays and the same laboratory test results, and reach differing conclusions on the most appropriate treatment. When your own well-being is involved, you owe it to yourself to get the best and most thorough medical advice possible.

If you want to avoid unnecessary surgery, ask the questions we have listed earlier—not only of your own doctor, but of the second physician from whom you seek an additional opinion. Have your medical records, x-rays and laboratory findings sent to the doctor(s) offering the second opinions. If your own physician can't or won't refer you to another doctor for a second opinion, you can contact a local medical school or hospital, your insurance company or your employer for a referral.

IS OUTPATIENT SURGERY AN OPTION?

At times, you may be able to avoid the hassles of hospitalization by having your surgery on an outpatient basis. More and more operations are being performed without the need for an overnight stay in the hospital. In a typical outpatient procedure, you arrive at the ambulatory surgery center—either a free-standing facility or part of a hospital—the morning of your operation, and within hours after surgery, you return home. This approach is much less costly than if you were admitted to the hospital and had to spend one or more nights there.

Some people find the thought of going home shortly after surgery a little unsettling at first. ("My mom had the same surgery ten years ago, and they kept her in the hospital for five days!") However, outpatient surgeries have become routine and generally pose no more risks than inpatient surgery.

A number of common surgical procedures can now be performed in ambulatory centers, including the following:

- Breast biopsy/lumpectomy
- Tubal ligation
- Dilation and curettage
- Cataract surgery
- Arthroscopic surgery
- Hernia repair
- Hemorrhoidectomy
- Tonsillectomy/adenoidectomy
- Vasectomy
- Cardiac catheterization
- Varicose vein removal
- Cosmetic surgery
- Excision of skin lesions

A number of studies have evaluated both cost and safety in outpatient procedures, comparing them with the same surgeries performed on patients admitted to the hospital. Consistently, this research has shown significant savings for operations performed in outpatient settings.

One study examined the use of arthroscopic knee surgery, in which only small incisions are made in the knee, through which the surgical instruments are carefully inserted for the operation. Patients undergoing this outpatient procedure were subjected to less preoperative testing and spent much less time at the outpatient facility than they would have at the hospital, including shorter periods in the operating room (mean operating time: 20 to 45 minutes less).

On occasion, you might undergo outpatient surgery, but either during or after the operation, your surgeon may decide to admit you to the hospital, perhaps because of a complication, or in order to observe you overnight. Even so, this is a relatively rare occurrence. Most outpatient procedures go according to plan, with patients finding them both convenient and economical. In 1992, the *New York Times* reported that among more than 22 million operations performed in U.S. hospitals in 1990, over half were conducted on an outpatient basis. That number is expected to grow rapidly, with outpatient surgeries increasing to nearly 70 percent of all surgeries by the year 2000.

"Minimally Invasive" Surgery—A Growing Trend

As an alternative to traditional "open" surgery, doctors now have the option in many cases of selecting "minimally invasive" surgery—operations that may require just small incisions and a short time in the operating room.

This technique is now being used by some surgeons for gallbladder operations, tubal ligations, appendectomies, hernia repairs and even for certain colon operations. It usually involves a tiny incision made in the skin, though which a thin, telescope-like instrument (a laparoscope) is inserted, allowing the surgeon to see into the area to be operated upon. The scalpel or other surgical instruments are then inserted through the same or another small incision, and the surgery itself is performed.

These procedures usually take less time than traditional surgery and involve briefer hospital stays. And there's more good news: Besides a quicker recovery for the patient, the cost of the hospital stay tends to be less than with more conventional operations.

However, one key point to keep in mind: Some of these procedures are relatively new. Be sure to select a surgeon who has a lot of experience with the operation you'll be having. Research shows the complication rate goes down with experience. Don't be afraid to ask how many times your surgeon has performed the operation. If it's a small number, find another doctor with more experience.

A few final thoughts: Choose the outpatient surgical facility as carefully as you select a hospital. Make sure that it is located near emergency facilities, just in case serious complications develop. Remember, no surgery is risk-free. And before agreeing to outpatient surgery, contact your insurance company to make certain it will pay for the procedure in this setting. Fortunately, most insurance companies now actually encourage the use of outpatient surgery because of the reduced costs.

GETTING THE MOST
FOR YOUR DENTAL DOLLAR

H ow much do you spend at your dentist's office each year? For most people, the cost of dental care is a relatively small portion of their overall health care expenses. They see their dentist only once or twice a year, and the cumulative bills for these visits are often modest compared to their annual doctors' bills. Nevertheless, many people feel anxious when they think of going to the dentist, and not just because they're afraid of the dental drill. It's because a large portion of dental expenses are paid directly out of their own pockets. In this chapter, we'll show you how to make the money you spend on dental care go as far as possible.

Who Pays for Dental Care?

In the best of all worlds, everyone would be protected by good medical and dental insurance. Unfortunately, too many Americans do not have dental insurance to fall back on. Employers often feel that they simply can't afford to offer their workers good dental coverage. After all, the cost of providing even the most basic medical insurance for their employees has risen to astronomical levels in recent years and, frankly, there just isn't much left in the benefits budget to cover dental care, too. When employers do offer dental insurance, it is frequently very limited.

As a result, many people check their bank balances first before deciding whether to see their dentist. These same individuals may schedule a doctor's appointment at the first sign of back pain or a sore throat—knowing that their health insurance will pay most or all of the medical bills. But they hesitate to see their dentist, even when they have a throbbing toothache or bleeding gums. If you're stretching to pay the regular bills, the out-of-pocket costs can make dental care seem like a "luxury" that can be put off until next week, next month—or indefinitely.

Who's Paying the Dentist's Bill?

On average, consumers end up paying about 20 percent of physicians' fees out-of-pocket, and 5 percent of the cost of hospitalization—while insurance companies and the government take care of the rest. But when it comes to dental care, more than half the cost comes out of our own wallets.

The problem is really twofold: (1) Far fewer people have dental insurance than have medical insurance; and (2) Insurance policies tend to provide far less comprehensive coverage for dental treatment than for medical care. Even the government provides only minimal protection for dental expenses through its programs for the elderly and the poor.

Here's what one study found about how dental services are paid for in the United States:

Total Cost of Dental Services $34 billion

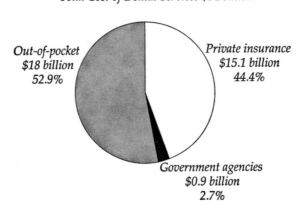

Out-of-pocket
$18 billion
52.9%

Private insurance
$15.1 billion
44.4%

Government agencies
$0.9 billion
2.7%

Source: Health Care Financing Administration, Office of the Actuary

Because of this reluctance to make visits to the dentist a priority, too many people receive little or no preventive dental care. When they do finally make their way into a dentist's chair, it is often to play "catch up"—treating a major problem that could have been cared for more easily (and less expensively) at an

> *One of the best ways to keep dental bills low is through regular dental examinations.*

earlier stage. For example, while your dentist may charge you $60 to fill a minor tooth cavity, it might cost you hundreds of dollars if you delay treatment until the condition deteriorates and you need a root canal instead.

Our message, then, is simple: One of the best ways to keep dental bills low is through regular dental examinations, even if the cost of these routine visits seems financially painful at the time. Of course, the very best way to eliminate dental problems altogether is through regular brushing and flossing.

Plan Ahead

Most people understand the importance of planning ahead to pay for the things they want or need. Whether they're saving for a vacation for themselves or to buy Christmas presents for loved ones, they find a way to set aside a little money until they've saved up the necessary funds.

You should make the same kind of commitment to your family's dental care. Just as you might put aside money each month to pay for part or all of your health insurance premiums, you need to budget for those twice-a-year dental checkups and cleanings, too. Anticipate your annual dental costs and build the projected expense into your family budget. Try depositing a few dollars each month into a savings account reserved just for dental care. With money already in this special "dental fund," you'll be less likely to put off making appointments with your dentist.

What About Dental Insurance?

Are you one of the lucky Americans who has dental insurance? If so, you probably receive it through a group plan offered by your employer, a labor union, or an association or organization to which you

Anticipate your annual dental costs and build the projected expense into your family budget.

belong. In most cases, group dental benefits are not part of the basic health coverage provided by employers, and usually require additional premium payments (sometimes, but rarely, covered in full by your employer).

Even if dental insurance is not available to you in a group plan, you still have some other options. Look into the individual dental policies offered by some insurance companies. But don't expect to find any bargains: As with other types of health insurance, individual dental plans tend to be more expensive than group coverage.

Whether you have a group or an individual policy, brace yourself for some inevitable loopholes. Read your policy carefully and you might find deductibles, co-insurance, limits on pre-existing conditions, and other factors that force you to share in the cost of your dental care—in addition to paying monthly premiums. For example, there may be a deductible, or a fixed amount that you have to pay out-of-pocket each year before the insurance company begins covering your dental expenses. It may be enough to make you wonder whether the insurance is worthwhile after all.

There is some good news: With dental insurance, if there's a deductible, it may be lower than you might find with medical insurance, as a way of encouraging you to seek preventive or early care before dental conditions worsen and become more expensive to treat. The same philosophy applies to co-insurance: Particularly with diagnostic and preventive services, your co-payments may be relatively low as an incentive for you to see your dentist regularly.

Because of the many possible limits on coverage, we urge you to read the insurance contract carefully when you're considering and comparing policies. Make sure you understand which services are covered, and which ones aren't. Dental plans vary considerably. For instance, does your policy cover only preventive services (basic examinations, cleaning, x-rays, fluoride treatments, sealants)? Or does it include major restorative care (such as bridges, crowns and root canals)? How about orthodontics? Are braces covered only for children, or are adults covered too? And are the cost of braces covered in all cases, or only when they're needed for other than cosmetic reasons?

What about reimbursement schedules in your dental plan? Are you responsible for paying 20 percent of your bills for *preventive* care under a co-insurance provision, but a larger portion (perhaps 50 percent) of more costly *restorative* procedures? Also, is there a waiting period for major services, requiring you to have the policy in force for 6 or 12 months before it will pay for care such as orthodontics? Checking the fine print in a policy now will eliminate surprises later when you get the bill from the dentist.

SERVICE PLANS

As you shop around for dental insurance, you may also encounter so-called "service" or "prepaid" dental plans. With this type of coverage, you (or your employer) will pay a flat premium or fee each month or quarter, and in return will receive dental services as defined in the policy. In many cases, you will be entitled to basic dental services (such as cleanings and fillings) at no additional charge, along with substantial coverage for major dental work (e.g., oral surgery, root canals). In some ways, these service plans are similar to HMOs, in that you make regular premium payments, for which you then receive most or all of your care.

This prepaid approach to dental care appeals to many people—but not all. Some are scared off by limitations that may be placed on their choice of dentists. With service plans, you usually need to choose from a list of dentists who have agreed to participate in the plan, and who will accept rates lower than those they might otherwise charge. Even so, because these service plans generally have cost advantages, many people are willing to give up their family dentist and begin seeing one of the dentists on the list.

As another alternative, you may choose to purchase a "discount dental plan." These plans charge "annual membership fees" rather than premiums. Members are eligible to receive dental services (including preventive care, oral surgery and orthodontics) at reduced rates. But again, the plan's own dentists must be used, and the plan administrator will provide you with a list of participating dentists to choose from in your area.

Let's look at the costs and services provided by two popular discount plans (the data are 1993 figures):

Montgomery Ward operates a discount program called the Signature Dental Plan. Its membership fee is $72 a year, which includes coverage for the family breadwinner and all financially dependent household members. For this annual charge, subscribers receive discounts on services ranging from diagnostic visits to braces and dentures. There is no charge for routine oral examinations. For more information, call (800) 346-0310.

Another discount program, called PlanPlus, is headquartered in Chicago. For a membership fee, heads of households and their immediate dependents receive discounts on preventive care, as well as on specialty treatment such as orthodontics, oral surgery, endodontics, periodontics and cosmetic dentistry. In addition to dental services, the plan also provides savings on many pharmacy items, as well as hearing and vision care. Members can purchase the entire plan for $89.95 or the dental plan only for $69.95. To reach PlanPlus, call (800) 424-3398.

Can You Really Save with a Discount Plan?

Discount dental plans are growing in popularity. In exchange for an annual "membership fee," these plans can provide considerable cost savings. Here's what certain dental services would have cost you out-of-pocket if you were a member of the Signature Dental Plan, compared to paying paying for the same services in full yourself. Keep in mind that these are 1992 prices, and can vary from one part of the country to another:

	Cost to Plan Member	Cost to Non-Member
Oral exam	$ 0	$ 28
Fluoride treatment	7	18
Sealant (per tooth)	12	23
Cleaning	25	39
Filling	40	58
Extraction	40	55
Root canal	210	278
Crown	350	476
Denture (upper or lower)	460	655
Braces	2,800	3,300

Source: Signature Dental Plan, 1992.

Although neither of these plans is available in all 50 states, you'll probably find several similar programs where you live. But, again, before sending in your membership fee, make sure you have read the fine print and know precisely what you're paying for.

> *Checking the fine print in a policy now will eliminate surprises later when you get the bill from the dentist.*

Other Sources of Low-Cost Care

If you're on an extremely tight budget, here's some good news: You don't have to forsake dental care completely. There are places you can turn to for low-cost dental treatment.

MEDICAID

First, what can you expect from the government? Frankly, very little. State Medicaid systems do provide some care, but it is not very extensive. Eligible children can receive certain dental treatment and, in some states, adults may be covered as well. Keep in mind, however, that because Medicaid is a state-operated program, the benefits vary from state to state. Also, in most cases, any dental care will have to be *preapproved* by Medicaid administrators. For complete information about the program in your state, call your local Medicaid office. And make sure your dentist will accept Medicaid's payment in full for services *before* you begin treatment.

MEDICARE

Medicare, a government-sponsored program designed primarily for those over 65, is not much help for most types of dental care. It may cover surgery of the jaw or its associated structures. It will probably also pay for the setting of a fracture of the jaw or facial bones. In short, Medicare will cover dental conditions that require hospitalization and that may make a *medical* condition worse; in such cases, treatment falls under Part A of Medicare, and hospitalization expenses would be covered once your deductible is paid. But when it comes to routine dental care, including fillings, tooth extractions or gum surgery, Medicare won't chip in at all. For more on Medicare, see Chapter 7.

DENTAL SCHOOL CLINICS

You may want to check out the dental school clinics in your area, which can be excellent sources of inexpensive dental services. You'll be cared for by dental students or residents (graduate dental students), whose work is closely monitored by the faculty of the dental school. Some people are hesitant to have students work on their teeth, no matter what the cost savings (The argument usually goes something like, "I don't want to be their guinea pig!"). However, keep in mind that these students are not only supervised by seasoned professionals, but they are often exposed to and are using cutting-edge technology and treatments. If you're not familiar with the location of the dental school nearest you, call hospitals in your area to see if they can refer you to a low-cost academic clinic.

DENTAL SOCIETY REFERRALS

There's still another way to find low-cost dental care. Contact your state or local dental society, which may tap the good will of its members to provide care at low fees, as well as offering services for homebound patients or those living in rural areas. Some of these programs provide low-cost, routine checkups and cleanings; others offer a more complete range of dental services. Some charge a nominal fee; others actually provide care at no cost. To determine the programs available in your community, and whether you and your family are eligible, call the dental societies directly.

Choosing a Dentist

No matter where you get your dental care, you will need to choose a dentist. Even if you belong to a service or prepaid dental plan, you will be given a choice of dentists from a list of participating professionals.

Most people spend much more time shopping for an automobile than they do for a dentist (or any other health care provider). It's important to choose your dentist carefully. Research the background of any dentist you're considering. Also, schedule a meeting with him or her before ever settling into the treatment chair. During this initial appointment, discuss the dentist's education and experience and find out the dentist's philosophy (for instance, how much emphasis is placed on preventive care, including home self-care). Ask if he or she will fully explain the diagnosis of any dental problems you may have, and any procedures that will be recommended. Also, check whether the dentist is available for dental emergencies.

During this initial meeting, you should also talk about fees and payment schedules. If you have dental insurance, make sure the dentist will accept it, and will follow any instructions built into your coverage (such as obtaining prior approval before going ahead with major procedures). And will the dentist's office submit the claim forms, or will that be your responsibility? Once you feel comfortable with your choice of a dentist, then schedule an appointment for actual care.

When you find a dentist you're happy with and who has proven his or her competence to you, stay put. By jumping from one dentist to another, you may jeopardize the continuity of your treatment, and perhaps increase its cost, too. However, if you become unhappy with the quality of your dentist's care or with the cost of services, remember that you're not bound to him or her. Ask friends and doctors for a referral to someone else. And keep in mind that in most states, you have the right to obtain copies of your dental records and x-rays, and have them sent to your new dentist. Yes, there may be a charge for

What Are the Dentist's Qualifications?

Find out as much as possible about a dentist before your first office visit. Here are sources that can help you learn more about a dentist:

- If you've been referred to the dentist by your primary care physician, an orthodontist, periodontist, or a friend or neighbor, ask him or her for as much background information about the dentist as possible, including impressions about the quality of work.

- Contact your state or local dental society. Ask if the dentist is a member, and for any information that's on file.

- Check the *American Dental Association Directory*, which compiles biographical listings of its members. This volume is available in many public libraries and all dental school libraries.

- Talk to faculty members at a nearby dental school.

> *Most people spend much more time shopping for an automobile than they do for a dentist.*

making copies of the x-rays, but don't let anyone tell you that you aren't entitled to those x-rays. The laws in most states say that you are.

Dental Products

There are many dental products on the market, from mouthrinses to electric toothbrushes to oral irrigators (e.g., Water Pik) to denture adhesives. The sheer number of choices available can be overwhelming, so let your dentist be your guide on what might be the most potent weapons in your personal campaign for healthy teeth. The American Dental Association's Council on Dental Materials, Instruments and Equipment awards its seal to those products that are deemed safe and effective, so items with this designation are generally good choices.

Be careful of unwarranted claims, however. As your dentist will probably tell you, irrigating devices do *not* get rid of plaque, although they may dislodge food particles that have become caught between your teeth. They might also be particularly helpful for people who wear orthodontic braces or who have bridges. But don't expect these devices to take the place of brushing and flossing. Talk to your dentist before using any dental device.

For More Information

In addition to your own dentist, the American Dental Association (ADA) is an excellent source of information about your dental health. The ADA may be able to answer your general questions, or put you in touch with someone who can. Write or call the ADA at the following address and phone number:

> Department of Public Information and Education
> American Dental Association
> 211 E. Chicago Avenue
> Chicago, IL 60611-2678
> (312) 440-2500

WHAT YOU NEED TO KNOW ABOUT MEDICARE

Do you think of America as a youthful nation? Most people do—but that's not what the statistics show. According to the U.S. Census Bureau, there are now more than 30 million Americans aged 65 and older. That's about ten times more senior citizens than there were at the turn of the 20th century. But just wait. With the baby-boom generation quickly aging—the first of the boomers will reach 65 in the year 2010—there is a geriatric explosion on the horizon. And that means more people will be turning to Medicare for coverage of their health care costs.

No matter what your own age, you need to know about Medicare. Even if your retirement is still decades away, it's not too early to begin thinking and planning for the future. And even if you are not yet eligible for Medicare yourself, you probably have a parent who is, or soon will be, and who may need some questions answered or some help in filling out forms.

What Is Medicare?

Medicare is a government health insurance program for people aged 65 or older (and for certain disabled people). It is run and supported financially by the federal government. While an agency called the Health Care Financing Administration establishes and implements Medicare policy, the administrative responsibilities of the program are delegated to private insurance companies (often called "intermediaries" or "carriers").

Since its founding in 1965, the Medicare program has become a key component in everyone's planning for old age. After all, as unpleasant as it may be to think about, illness tends to occur much more frequently in the elderly than in the young. And were it not for Medicare, many older Americans would find their health care bills an overwhelming burden tarnishing their golden years. In its first year, the Medicare program cost the federal government a little over $3 billion. In 1990, that figure had soared to $109 billion!

But before you think that at age 65, you can breathe a sigh of relief—("Finally, the government is going to take care of all my medical bills!")—think again. Medicare was never intended to cover *all* the medical expenses of the elderly. In fact, you may be surprised to learn that you *will* have out-of-pocket health care costs in your old age, perhaps even substantial ones. There's no argument over that.

A TWO-PART PROGRAM

The Medicare program consists of two parts. Later in this chapter, we'll describe them in more detail. For now, let's briefly get acquainted with them:

Part A covers a portion of the cost of hospitalization, as well as expenses for inpatient skilled nursing homes, hospice care and some other health-related services. You'll receive Part A automatically and without charge when you turn 65, if you're also eligible for Social Security.

Part B covers a portion of other medical expenses, primarily doctors' and surgeons' bills, as well as some outpatient services (such as emergency room care, x-rays, laboratory tests and certain prescription medications). Part B is an optional feature of the program, and requires those who sign up for it to pay a monthly premium.

Keep in mind that if you decide that you just want coverage for the most expensive care, generally hospital treatment, you can sign up for only Part A. However, if you want more comprehensive protection (which may become increasingly important with advancing age), it makes sense to accept the plan in its entirety, both Parts A and B. That's what we recommend for most people.

An important note: You need to remember that even if you're covered by both parts of Medicare, it will not pay all your medical expenses.

For instance, there is a deductible and a co-payment (or co-insurance) provision in both parts of the program, as well as a monthly premium for Part B. Consequently, in these times of rising costs, many senior citizens are having to dig deeper into their savings to cover the cost of their medical services.

> *You need to remember that even if you're covered by both parts of Medicare, it will not pay all your medical expenses.*

As you might guess, this is a disturbing and stressful situation for people who are often already living on limited, fixed incomes; many fear that if a single, serious illness strikes, they could lose everything. Even so, if you plan ahead and protect yourself with supplemental insurance coverage, you won't have to worry about how the bills are going to get paid. Later in this chapter, we'll show you how to ensure that you are well protected. If you follow our guidelines, you can have peace of mind in your later years.

Do You Qualify for Medicare?

The day you reach age 65, you will become eligible for Medicare *if* you already qualify for Social Security benefits (or Railroad Retirement benefits) based on your previous wage earnings and tax payments. If either you or your spouse worked long enough (generally ten years or more), you are probably eligible for both Social Security and Medicare.

Besides spouses, other people may qualify for benefits that are contingent on the Social Security account of someone close to them who has met the working requirements: This includes widows and widowers, as well as ex-spouses from a marriage that lasted for at least ten years and who have not remarried. You might also claim benefits if you are a parent who received support from an adult child who qualified for Social Security, and who is now disabled or has died.

In addition, if you are disabled yourself, Medicare may be able to help you. There are special guidelines that will allow you to enter the Medicare program, even if you're under 65. Specifically, you must have received Social Security disability benefits for at least 24 months. You might qualify for other reasons, as well: For example, if you require ongoing dialysis treatments because of permanent kidney failure, or if you are a kidney transplant recipient. In these cases, you might also be eligible for Medicare benefits, no matter what your age. (For more information about these special circumstances, contact your local Social Security office.)

Some people, of course, won't fall into any of the above categories. Let's say that you are at least 65 years old but are not eligible for Social Security, and so cannot automatically participate in Medicare. If that's your situation, don't worry. You won't be shut out completely. You *can* receive Part A of Medicare, although you will have to pay a monthly premium to do so, just as you would with any other insurance policy. And, like all other Medicare recipients, you'll also be eligible to enroll in Part B, paying the same premium for Part B as everyone else.

Are You Eligible? A Quick Review

You qualify for Medicare if you meet any of the following criteria:

- You are 65 years old or over, and are eligible for Social Security based on your work record. You'll receive Part A of Medicare without paying a premium.

- If you are 65 or over and do not have enough work credits to qualify for Medicare, you can receive Part A benefits by paying a monthly premium.

- You are disabled and have been receiving Social Security disability for 24 months. You automatically qualify for Part A of Medicare without being charged a monthly premium.

- You are the spouse of a Social Security-eligible individual—or are the widow or widower of such an individual. You can obtain Part A of Medicare without paying premiums.

- In all of the above cases, you can also receive Part B of Medicare, but in each instance, you are required to pay a monthly premium to participate.

How to Apply for Medicare

The government actually makes your participation in Medicare quite easy. If you already qualify for and are receiving Social Security benefits upon turning 65, you will automatically be enrolled in Part A. It's that easy! No additional Medicare application is needed, at least for Part A. However, you will receive a Medicare card in the mail, asking you to decide whether you want to participate in Part B, as well. Make your decision, and follow the instructions on the card if you choose to enroll. If you don't receive this application, call your nearest Social Security office and request one.

If you qualify for but have not yet begun receiving Social Security benefits when you turn 65 (for example, if you work right up to your 65th birthday), you'll have to file an application for Medicare. However, you need to keep some deadlines in mind. First and foremost, you should apply as early as possible to avoid delays in your coverage. By joining during your "initial enrollment period," you'll avoid penalties for late sign-up. How long does this initial enrollment period last? It extends for seven months, beginning three months before the month in which you first qualify for Medicare. Thus, if you will turn 65 on July 1, 1995, your initial enrollment period starts three months *before* your birthday—on April 1 of that year—and ends seven months from April 1—on November 1.

Remember: *It is to your advantage to sign up during the first three months of your initial enrollment period.* You won't be shut out of the program if you let it pass by. However, there may be delays in beginning your Part B coverage. Rather than starting during the month you celebrate your 65th birthday, your coverage may be delayed from one to three months. And what if you become sick in the interim? You could be left holding a stack of medical bills for which you could have been covered, but aren't.

At times, people neglect to sign up for Part B during the entire seven-month initial enrollment period. The sign-up period comes and goes, and they haven't taken any action. Even then, however, their opportunities aren't gone forever, although they may have to wait several months for a "general enrollment period" to arrive. New sign-ups for Part B can occur during these times, which take place during the first three months of every year—that is, from January 1 to March 31. However, if you join the program during one of these general enrollment periods, brace yourself (and your pocketbook) for some bad news: You'll have to pay a penalty because of your tardiness. The government will raise your Part B premiums about ten percent for each 12 months you delayed your enrollment. Over the years, that could add up to a lot of money.

Incidentally, if you're one of those people we mentioned earlier who does not meet the requirements for premium-free Part A insurance but still decides to buy into the Medicare system, you can sign up for Part A during either an initial or a general enrollment period—although, again, the earlier the better. Remember that, in your case, you'll be paying monthly premiums for Part A, just as you will for Part B. And if you enroll at the earliest possible time, you can avoid stiff premium penalties; late enrollment in Part A may cause an increase in your premiums of as much as ten percent if you sign up more than a year after you first become eligible for the program. Thus, the longer you wait before enrolling, the more costly your coverage will become. Keep these penalties to a minimum, or eliminate them completely, by enrolling early.

SPECIAL CIRCUMSTANCES

By now, you should have determined which of the above situations apply to you. For some people, however, there may be additional, special circumstances that bear on their enrollment in Medicare.

What if you decide that you'd prefer not to participate in Medicare, at least not yet? For instance, even though you are 65 years old, you may still be working and be covered under your employer's health plan. (In fact, if you work for a firm that has 20 or more employees, you *must* be offered the same company medical benefits as younger employees.)

If you feel that's all the coverage you need, you can delay enrollment in Medicare without having a penalty eventually added to your Part B premium. At some point, perhaps when you finally retire or if your company goes out of business, you can then join the government insurance program during a special enrollment period. When that occurs, the penalty should be waived; if it isn't, contact the Social Security office, letting the plan administrators know that you had been covered by an employer's health plan when you were first eligible for Medicare, and postponed your enrollment for that reason.

Incidentally, are you curious why the federal government encourages you to sign up for Medicare as early as possible, and usually imposes penalties when you delay? There is some logic to these stipulations. Medicare officials simply don't want millions of people signing up only when they become ill, thus

> *While most people think of Part A of Medicare as hospitalization insurance, it goes well beyond covering just hospital costs.*

burdening the system with huge expenses at the time of enrollment. Rather, they'd prefer to have you join when you first become eligible at age 65, and perhaps pass through some relatively healthy years of paying Part B premiums before you begin making significant claims. It's a way to try to keep the system solvent.

A Closer Look at Your Medical Coverage

As we've already seen, Medicare is composed of two parts. Together, they provide you with coverage for hospitalization, doctors' fees and other health care expenses. Let's examine the scope of your Medicare coverage more closely:

MEDICARE PART A

So you can understand how Part A works, let's look at some of the provisions that help determine how much of your medical expenses the government will pay—and how much will be left for you to cover out of your own pocket.

BENEFIT PERIOD

Your Medicare protection is linked to "benefit periods." They help the government calculate the medical services you utilize that qualify under the Medicare system.

Here are the most important elements about benefit periods to bear in mind: After you join Medicare, your first benefit period begins the day you are admitted to a hospital. It ends 60 consecutive days after your discharge from either the hospital or a skilled nursing home (if you were transferred to the nursing home following your hospitalization).

After one benefit period ends, another one begins the next time you are hospitalized. With each new benefit period, you start with a clean slate, and are awarded a new set of Medicare benefits.

Within each benefit period, there are some limitations and some responsibilities that you have to assume. For example:

- You must pay a new deductible in each benefit period. In 1994, that deductible is $696, meaning that you are responsible for the first $696 of covered hospital expenses before the government begins reimbursing the hospital for services. That's a sizable chunk of money, but the government believes the deductible is necessary in order to keep the overall costs of Medicare under control.

- Once you have met the deductible, Medicare will pay your expenses in full for up to 60 days of hospitalization.

- If you have a prolonged illness and your hospitalization lasts beyond 60 days, then you must begin paying a portion of your

The Fine Print . . .

Several conditions must be met in order for Medicare to pay for your inpatient hospital care. If these circumstances are not applicable to your medical situation, you will not be covered. The conditions include:

- A doctor must prescribe inpatient hospital care for treatment of your illness or injury.

- The care you require can be provided only in the hospital.

- The hospital is a formal participant in the Medicare program.

- Your stay in the hospital has not been disapproved by review panels—for instance, the Utilization Review Committee of the hospital, a Peer Review Organization or a Medicare intermediary.

hospital bill each day for the next 30 days—that is, from days 61 through 90. The portion of your bill that you are responsible for is called "co-insurance" or "co-payment." In 1994, this co-insurance amounts to $174 per day, which you'd be billed for directly by the hospital. Medicare pays the remainder of the bill beyond the initial $174 each day.

- After 90 days in the hospital, you are required to pay the entire cost of your continued hospitalization yourself—with one exception. During your lifetime, you are entitled to 60 "reserve days," which you may apply to any benefit period in which your hospitalization goes beyond 90 days. During these reserve days, Medicare will help cover the cost of your hospitalization, but you must pay a larger portion of your daily hospital bill than the usual $174 co-payment. (In 1994, you're responsible for paying $348 for each reserve day). Don't forget that 60 days is your limit. Once these reserve days are gone, you can't get a new supply. Thus, if you use 12 reserve days during one hospitalization, you will have only 48 reserve days remaining over your lifetime. Once they are used up, you must start paying your hospital expenses in full for any hospitalization over 90 days.

Let's look at a typical scenario to help you better understand how a benefit period works:

Charles enrolled in Medicare on January 1. He had heart disease, and as his condition worsened, he was admitted to the hospital for the first time on May 1. Discharged on May 8, he used seven days of his initial benefit period. The hospital billed him $696—the deductible for his Medicare covered expenses—and the rest of the bill was paid by Medicare.

Two weeks later, on May 22, Charles' condition took a turn for the worse. His doctor decided to readmit him to the hospital. Because 60 days had not passed between hospitalizations, Charles' care fell under the same benefit period, and the first day of this new hospitalization was counted as the eighth day of hospital care in his original benefit period. Since this hospitalization was considered a continuation of the same benefit period, Charles did not have to pay another deductible. This time, he remained in the hospital for a week, returning home on May 29.

Then, on August 15, Charles became seriously ill again. In this instance, however, more than 60 days had passed since he was last hospitalized. Thus, a new Medicare benefit period began, meaning that he became responsible for paying a new hospital deductible. As he did during his first hospitalization, he had to pay the initial $696 of covered services for this second benefit period.

PART A: HOW BROAD IS YOUR COVERAGE?

While most people think of Part A of Medicare as hospitalization insurance, it goes well beyond covering just hospital costs. Listed below are the kinds of services for which Part A offers protection.

Part A of Medicare helps pay for four kinds of care when they are deemed medically necessary:

1. Inpatient hospital care
2. Inpatient care in a skilled nursing facility
3. Home health care
4. Hospice care

INPATIENT HOSPITAL CARE

Medicare pays for your inpatient hospital care. Here are the specific services covered under Part A:

- A semiprivate room
- Meals
- Regular nursing services
- Cost of special care units, such as intensive care
- Drugs supplied by the hospital while you are a patient
- Blood transfusions (except charges for the first three pints)
- Laboratory tests that are listed on your hospital bill
- X-rays and other radiology services
- Medical supplies such as casts, surgical dressings and splints

- Operating and recovery room expenses
- Rehabilitation services such as physical therapy, occupational therapy and speech pathology
- Use of appliances, such as wheelchairs

Some services are excluded from coverage under Part A. They include:

- Items that you might ask to have in your hospital room for the sake of convenience or enjoyment, such as a telephone or a television set
- Private duty nurses
- Extra charges for a private hospital room, unless your doctor considers it to be a medical necessity

SKILLED NURSING FACILITY CARE

These days, hospitals are discharging patients sooner than ever before. If you've been in a hospital lately, you might have felt that the doctors and nurses were more interested in getting you out of the hospital than in getting you well. That's an exaggeration, of course, but as patients are being released sooner, skilled nursing home services are becoming a more important component of health care for many Americans.

Here's the bottom line: Even when you're ready to leave the hospital, you may not be well enough to go home. So as you continue to recover, you could need the help of nursing care provided or supervised by licensed nurses.

Talk to your doctor before you are discharged from the hospital. He or she may advise you to go to a nursing facility, which can serve as a transition on your way home. Some nursing homes deliver fairly intensive care, or *skilled* care; many others, however, provide only unskilled or custodial care, which just helps individuals with the tasks of daily living (such as eating, bathing, getting in and out of bed, walking and taking medications).

If your doctor recommends temporary care in a skilled nursing facility, some of your worries about costs will be over. Many services in a skilled nursing home are covered under Part A of Medicare. Even so, make sure you understand the type of care that is and isn't included in your protection. You might think, "If I'm in a nursing home, that's

As patients are being released sooner, skilled nursing home services are becoming a more important component of health care for many Americans.

all the government wants to know." In fact, there are specific guidelines that must be met before Medicare will pay.

Here's what you need to know: Part A will pay for only a limited nursing home stay—and *only* in a skilled nursing facility. Longer stays (even in skilled nursing facilities) and custo-dial care are *not* provided for under Medicare. At a skilled nursing facility, here is what Part A will cover:

- A semiprivate room
- Meals
- Routine nursing services
- Rehabilitation services, such as physical, occupational and speech therapy
- Medications provided by the nursing facility
- Blood transfusions (except for charges for the first three pints)
- Medical supplies (e.g., casts and splints)
- The use of wheelchairs, walkers and other appliances

Even in a skilled nursing facility, some of the care you receive is *not* covered by Part A, including:

- Special items of convenience that you ask for, such as a television set or a telephone in your room
- Additional fees for a private room, unless your doctor certifies that private quarters are required for medical reasons
- The care you receive from your doctor when you are in the nursing facility (Part B of Medicare covers these doctor's bills)
- Private-duty nursing care

For each benefit period, Medicare will pay for a maximum of 100 days in a skilled nursing facility. The first 20 days will be covered in full by Part A. After that, you will need to pay daily co-insurance during the next 80 days (days 21 to 100); in 1994, that co-payment is $87.00 a day. Beyond 100 days, Medicare's responsibility ends, and you must assume the full cost of any additional days.

Skilled Nursing Care: How to Be Sure You Qualify

If you receive care in a skilled nursing facility, Part A of Medicare will help pay for that care if all of the following conditions are met:

- A doctor certifies that you need *daily* skilled nursing or skilled rehabilitation care (such as physical therapy). If you need this care only occasionally—perhaps just once or twice a week—Part A of Medicare will *not* pay for your nursing home services.

- The nursing home selected must formally participate in Medicare as a skilled nursing facility. (This is a very important point; most nursing homes in the U.S. are *not* skilled nursing facilities and do not participate in the program. Ask the business office at the nursing facility you are considering if it participates in Medicare, or ask your local Social Security office to find out for you by checking directly with the Health Care Financing Administration.)

- You must have been a patient in a hospital for at least three consecutive days (not counting the day you were discharged), and have been admitted to the nursing facility shortly after you checked out of the hospital (usually within 30 days). If you receive care in a nursing facility, return home, but then need to return to the nursing facility within 30 days, a new three-day stay in the hospital is unnecessary in order for Medicare to continue paying for that skilled nursing care.

- Your care in the skilled nursing home must be for the same medical problem that you were treated for in the hospital, or for a condition that developed while you were in the nursing facility.

- A Medicare reviewer or intermediary (an individual assigned by the government to help administer the Medicare program) must not rule that your stay in a skilled nursing home is unnecessary.

HOME HEALTH CARE

After a hospital stay, there are times when you may not need to be admitted to a nursing facility, although you still might require some help at home. That's when home health services can be important. Some of them are even covered by Part A of Medicare.

Home health care generally involves periodic visits to your home by a health care professional—perhaps for 30 to 60 minutes, several times a week—to provide skilled nursing care, physical and speech therapy, and other treatments. This care might include changing dressings on wounds, giving injections or setting up intravenous medications. The skilled medical professionals (e.g., nurses, physical therapists) who specialize in and provide these services typically work for businesses called home health agencies.

Here are the home health services provided under Medicare Part A:

- Part-time skilled nursing care
- Physical therapy
- Speech therapy

If you need any of the above services, Medicare will also cover the following:

- Occupational therapy (for example, learning to do everyday tasks such as dressing oneself)
- Part-time services provided by home health aides
- Health care supplies
- Medical social services
- Durable medical equipment such as wheelchairs, walkers and oxygen equipment (80 percent of the cost)

Part A will *not* pay for certain home health services, including:

- Around-the-clock private-duty nursing
- Medications
- Food and meals delivered to you at home
- Homemaking or personal services (such as cooking, cleaning, laundry or grocery shopping)
- Blood transfusions

So how extensive is Part A's reimbursement for covered services? It may sound too good to be true, but Medicare pays their complete approved cost, requiring *no* co-payment for most services.

There is one exception to this comprehensive coverage: As noted above, you are responsible for a 20 percent co-payment on any durable medical equipment you might need. And, of course, you must also pay in full for any home services that are not covered by Medicare.

Just a word about one other benefit with home health services: Don't worry about taking care of the needed paperwork yourself. The home health agency will fill out and submit the necessary forms and bills.

HOSPICE CARE

In recent years, there has been a growing availability of hospice care. This is a special type of service—often providing mostly pain relief and supportive care—for people who are terminally ill with a disease such as cancer or AIDS.

Meeting the Criteria for Home Services

Although Medicare will pay for home services, all of the following conditions must first be met:

- You must be confined to your home.

- You must be under a doctor's care, and he or she must decide that you require home health care. The doctor must arrange for a personalized home health plan for you, order the services, and review your care plan periodically.

- The care you require should be *part-time* skilled nursing care, or physical or speech therapy.

- The home health agency that provides your care must be certified to participate in Medicare. Make sure your doctor refers you to a participating agency, and ask that agency to determine whether the services you need will qualify for Medicare reimbursement. You should not be billed for this evaluation.

Although Part A covers hospice care, certain circumstances must be met:

- A physician must confirm that the patient really is terminally ill.

- The patient must decide to accept hospice care rather than standard Medicare benefits.

- The hospice itself must be a participant in the Medicare program.

Although "benefit periods" are utilized in hospice care, they have characteristics unique to this aspect of the program. Medicare will provide coverage for two 90-day periods, followed by a 30-day period; if necessary, an extension period of indefinite length can also be utilized. While these benefit periods can be used successively, one after the other, they can also be spaced out as needed.

When it comes to hospice care, Part A covers all Medicare-covered services without the need for the patient to pay any deductible. A small co-payment is required, however, for outpatient medications and inpatient respite care. (Respite care is a short inpatient stay to provide a temporary break for the usual caregiver.) Under the co-insurance provision, you are responsible for five percent or $5 for each prescription drug, whichever is less. For respite services, the co-payment is five percent.

During hospice care, patients sometimes require treatment for a medical problem not directly associated with their terminal condition. If that happens, Medicare will provide needed services under the traditional Medicare program. Let's say, for instance, that an individual is receiving hospice care for terminal colon cancer; during this time, he slips on a throw rug and breaks his hip. The Medicare program would cover treatment for the hip injury under the traditional Parts A and B of Medicare.

MEDICARE PART B

Part B is the optional portion of Medicare that is supported by premium payments from those who choose to subscribe to it. Although its primary emphasis is upon paying for doctors' services, Part B coverage is broader than that. Here's what else your premium dollars pay for: outpatient hospital care (including emergency room services),

diagnostic tests, durable medical equipment, ambulance services, and certain
other services and supplies. We'll describe
this coverage in more detail in a moment.

> *When it comes to hos-
> pice care, Part A covers
> all Medicare-covered
> services without the
> need for the patient to
> pay any deductible.*

Most people look at the scope of Part B
coverage, and figure they've got to have
it—if they can afford it. In the majority of
cases, that's a wise decision. And how
much does it cost? In 1994, Part B premi-
ums are $41.10 a month. Compared to what you'd pay for similar
coverage in the private sector, it's actually a bargain. If you do
become a Part B subscriber, your monthly premium will be deducted
from your Social Security check or, if you don't receive Social
Security benefits yet, you will be billed at regular intervals.

However, as with Part A of Medicare, you will have certain out-of-
pocket expenses associated with Part B, most notably an annual
deductible and co-payments. The Part B deductible is $100 in 1994.
This means you are responsible for the first $100 in covered,
approved expenses each year before your Medicare protection kicks
in and begins paying benefits. The deductible can be met by any combination of covered services—that is, if you pay $50 for a doctor's bill
and $50 for blood tests, you will have satisfied your Part B deductible
for the year; you need not pay a separate deductible in each category
of medical services.

Even so, once you have reached your deductible, it's not time to celebrate yet. You still have some financial obligations under Part B in the
form of co-insurance or a co-payment which requires you to pay a
portion—usually 20 percent of the approved amount—of most of
your remaining bills under Part B.

Thus, there's no "free lunch" when it comes to Part B. On the other
hand, if you have no other health coverage, we believe Part B is
something you should seriously consider. Of course, if you're one of
those people who's still working after the age of 65, your employee
health benefits might be all the coverage you need. But if you're
retired and you tried to buy this kind of coverage from a private
insurance company, your premiums would be very high—if you
could obtain the coverage at all in your age category.

Which Outpatient Services Are Covered Under Part B?

If you have no other health coverage, we believe Part B is something you should seriously consider.

A wide variety of outpatient hospital and medical services are covered by Part B of Medicare. After meeting your annual deductible, Medicare will reimburse you for 80 percent of the approved cost of the following services:

- Treatment in an emergency room

- Services in an outpatient facility, including "same day surgery"

- Lab tests and x-rays billed by a hospital

- Blood transfusions given in outpatient settings

- Kidney dialysis

- Mental health care in a partial hospitalization psychiatric program, if a physician confirms that without it, inpatient care would be needed. (Some treatment for mental illness outside the hospital may also be covered.)

- Medical supplies such as splints and casts

- Medications that cannot be self-administered

- Outpatient occupational, physical and speech therapy

- Diagnostic tests: When you undergo diagnostic tests, Part B will pay the approved fee for many of them in full, as long as they are conducted by certified laboratories that participate in the Medicare program. These labs can be independent facilities, part of a hospital outpatient department, or located in a doctor's own office. Before undergoing tests, ask whether the lab has received Medicare approval to perform them.

Some screening tests are also covered by Part B. For instance, Medicare will help pay for Pap tests every three years, and more often for women who are considered at high risk (because of factors such as a family history of cervical cancer). Mammograms to screen for breast cancer are also included in covered services; to find out how often Medicare will pay for mammograms, contact your Medicare carrier.

- Ambulance Transportation: Although ambulance services are covered under Part B, certain conditions must be met. For instance, it must be clear that if other types of transportation are used instead, your well-being might be jeopardized. Coverage is also provided only to or from your house and a hospital or skilled nursing home (not a doctor's office). The ambulance, as well as its personnel and equipment, must meet Medicare standards.

Part B will not cover certain outpatient services, such as routine physical exams, most foot and eye care, many immunizations, and ear exams conducted for the purpose of prescribing hearing aids.

Does Medicare Part B cover alternative types of health care? Many people get at least part of their health care from practitioners other than a doctor of medicine or a doctor of osteopathy. But when the creators of Part B put together the program, they weren't very generous in including the services of these other practitioners. Just scan the box on page 164 describing some of the exclusions from Part B coverage. You may not think these limitations are fair, but you'll receive reimbursement for only a limited number of services administered by certain health care providers. For example:

Chiropractors: Chiropractic care is not covered by Medicare, with one exception: Manual manipulation of the spine to care for a subluxation that an x-ray has identified.

Podiatrists: Medicare *will* kick in to help pay for podiatric services to treat injuries or diseases of the foot, such as bunion deformities or ingrown toenails. However, more commonplace, hygienic care by a podiatrist, such as treatment of corns and calluses or nail trimming, is not covered. (Note: If you need foot care because you have a disease such as diabetes, this care—whether by a podiatrist, osteopath or medical doctor—*is* covered by Medicare.)

Dentists: Forget about Medicare coverage for routine dental treatment, such as fillings, extractions, root canals or tooth replacements. The only help you'll receive from Part B is if the dental problem involves more than just the teeth and gums (for example, a fracture of the jaw).

Optometrists: Medicare will not cover routine eye exams, and in most cases, will not pay for eyeglasses or contact lenses. Following cataract surgery, however, Medicare will open up its coffers a little, covering the cost of cataract eyeglasses, contact lenses or intraocular lenses.

WHEN ARE A DOCTOR'S CHARGES "APPROVED"?

You've read that Medicare pays 80 percent of the "approved" charge for care under Part B. You might have wondered, "What charges are 'approved'?"

This can be confusing, but it's really not that complicated. It was instituted as a cost-control effort, and here's how it works:

Medicare will not necessarily pay its 80 percent share of doctors' bills based on what your doctor charges. Instead, it has created its own fee schedule, which assigns a particular payment schedule to given services—a so-called "reasonable charge"—taking into consideration factors such as variations in the cost of practicing medicine in different parts of the country. This "approved" charge is frequently less than the amount billed by the doctor; he or she may charge $75 for a service, but Medicare has "approved" it at $60. When that's the case, the government will pay only 80 percent of the *approved* figure, not the actual charge. And guess who's responsible for the rest?

For example, let's say that your doctor has billed you $75 for an office visit, but in evaluating this service, Medicare notices that its "approved" amount is only $55. This means Medicare will pay 80 percent of $55 (.80 x $55 = $44), and you are responsible for the remainder (the co-payment), or $31!

This is probably a much bigger bill than you expected. But this does not always happen, and that's because many doctors have begun to accept Medicare "assignment"—that is, they agree to accept Medicare's approved amount as total payment for a particular service. In the example above, although your doctor's usual fee might be $75, he would agree to accept a $55 "assignment" since you are a Medicare patient. In this particular instance, after Medicare pays your doctor $44 (its 80 percent portion), you will be billed for the remaining $11. Once you write a check for your $11 co-payment, the bill will be considered paid in full.

You can save money by going to doctors who accept assignment. But how do you find out if a particular doctor has agreed to this Medicare-approved amount? It's easier than you think. You can obtain a free directory of these doctors by contacting the Medicare carrier in your area. It's called the *Medicare-Participating Physician/Supplier Directory*, and doctors are given the opportunity to sign participation agreements—and thus appear in the directory—every year. You can also look at a copy of the directory at your local Social Security office.

One other important point: There still are doctors who believe that Medicare's fixed reimbursement rates are unfairly low, and have decided *not* to accept assignment. If you choose to go to one of them anyway, even if it costs you more out-of-pocket, keep in mind that even these doctors have a limit on how much they can bill you. Remember the example above, where you had to write your doctor a check for $31 for a $75 service. Well, that actually can't happen anymore. As of 1993, these physicians can charge Medicare patients no more than 115 percent of Medicare's approved fees. So, if Medicare has decided on $150 as the approved fee for a particular procedure, doctors can charge you no more than $172.50—or 115 percent of the approved figure. Of course, these same physicians can charge their non-Medicare patients more if they choose; they are only limited in what they can charge Medicare patients.

If you believe you have been billed too much, complain to your doctor and ask for an adjustment on your charges. If you have already paid the bill, request a refund.

What About a Second Opinion?

In some instances, surgery is the best treatment for a serious medical condition. But that isn't always the case. There is increasing evidence that many operations are unnecessary, and that patients can often be treated just as well in less invasive—and less expensive—ways. For that reason, Medicare's message is simple: Get a second opinion before going ahead with any surgical procedure.

As an incentive, Medicare will pay for 80 percent of the approved cost of obtaining that second opinion (assuming that your annual deductible has already been met). If the first and second doctors do not agree

Doctors' Services: What's Covered, What's Not

If you're looking for peace of mind, Part B coverage can certainly give you some, even though there are certain gaps in the protection. When it comes to doctors' services, here's the type of coverage you can expect:

- Medical and surgical services, whether received in the physician's office, a hospital, a nursing home, or even in your own home
- Diagnostic tests and procedures that are part of your treatment
- Radiology and pathology services provided by doctors (while you are a hospital inpatient or outpatient)
- Mental health services (coverage is limited)
- Other services:
    - —X-rays
    - —Drugs that cannot be self-administered
    - —Care by a nurse in your doctor's office
    - —Blood (and blood component) transfusions
    - —Medical supplies
    - —Physical and occupational therapy, and speech pathology services

Services provided by your doctor that are *not* insured by Part B:

- Routine physical examinations
- Tests that are part of these routine examinations (although some Pap tests and mammograms are covered)
- Most routine foot care
- Most dental treatment
- Examinations conducted in order to prescribe or fit eyeglasses or hearing aids
- Routine immunizations (exceptions: pneumococcal vaccines and hepatitis B immunizations for people at high risk are covered)
- Cosmetic surgery (although coverage is allowed if the surgery is necessary because of an accidental injury or to improve the ability of a malformed body part to function)

on whether surgery is really necessary, Medicare encourages you to get
even a third opinion, for which it will
also pay 80 percent.

Many doctors have begun to accept Medicare "assignment"—that is, they agree to accept Medicare's approved amount as total payment for a particular service.

If you have questions about second
opinions, the Medicare program has
set up a telephone hotline to respond
to your inquiries. The numbers for
this Second Surgical Opinion Hotline
are: 800-638-6833; 800-492-6603 (in Maryland).

By contacting the Medicare carrier in your area, you can also obtain
names of nearby doctors who will give you second opinions, or
receive a referral to an organization that can do so.

Medicare Prepayment Plans: Is One Right for You?

If you're interested in saving money—and who isn't?—you might
consider joining a managed care or prepayment plan. A growing
number of these plans have signed contracts with the federal government to provide services to Medicare beneficiaries. If you join one of
these plans, it must provide at a minimum all the services offered in
the Medicare guidelines. In many cases, it will offer even more.

How do these programs work for Medicare patients? When you join
a prepayment program, Medicare will begin to pay a monthly premium to the HMO or other plan, which will cover most of the costs for
your care. At the same time, however, you may be obligated to pay
the HMO small additional premium payments; you might also be
responsible for limited co-payments for certain services.

Overall, you will often come out ahead with an HMO: Your out-of-
pocket expenses will tend to be lower and much more predictable
than with a traditional fee-for-service Medicare plan. Many people
find it easier to budget their health care costs with an HMO, since
they are dealing with fixed payments that cover all or nearly all of
their care. And they probably won't have to invest in supplemental
private health insurance (Medigap), which we'll describe in the last
major section of this chapter.

> *If you believe you have been billed too much, complain to your doctor and ask for an adjustment on your charges.*

To enroll in a prepayment plan, you must meet several requirements:

- You must live in the area served by the plan.
- You also must enroll and maintain your participation in Part B of Medicare.
- You must not be obtaining care in a Medicare-certified hospice.
- You must not be entitled to Medicare due to kidney failure.

If joining an HMO sounds intriguing, you might choose to give it a try. If you turn out to be dissatisfied with your care or any other aspect of the prepaid plan, you can withdraw from it and immediately enroll in the fee-for-service Medicare program.

Keep in mind one important limitation with HMOs: If you enroll in one, you will have to obtain *all* your health care from that organization. You won't have a choice of outside doctors and hospitals. True, you could occasionally get services elsewhere, but in those cases, you will have to pay for this care out of your own pocket, since neither the HMO nor Medicare will cover these costs (except for emergency treatment).

FINDING AN HMO

There is an easy way to find out if any HMOs in your community have contracted with the Medicare program. Simply call the office listed below that corresponds to the state in which you live:

In Connecticut, Maine, Massachusetts, New Hampshire, Rhode Island and Vermont: Beneficiary Services Branch; 617-565-1232

In New York, New Jersey, Puerto Rico and the Virgin Islands: Carrier Operations Branch; 212-264-8522

In Delaware, District of Columbia, Maryland, Pennsylvania, Virginia and West Virginia: Beneficiary Services Branch; 215-596-1332

In Alabama, Florida, Georgia, Kentucky, Mississippi, North Carolina, South Carolina and Tennessee: HMO Branch; 404-331-2549

In Illinois, Indiana, Michigan, Minnesota, Ohio and Wisconsin: HMO Branch; 312-353-7180

In Arkansas, Louisiana, New Mexico, Oklahoma and Texas: Beneficiary Services Branch; 214-767-6401

In Iowa, Kansas, Missouri and Nebraska: Program Services Branch; 816-426-2866

In Colorado, Montana, North Dakota, South Dakota, Utah and Wyoming: Beneficiary Services Branch; 303-844-4024, ext. 238

In American Samoa, Arizona, California, Guam, Hawaii and Nevada: Beneficiary Services Branch; 415-744-3617

In Alaska, Idaho, Oregon and Washington: Beneficiary Services Branch; 206-553-0800.

What If There's an Error?

Whether you're using your Medicare benefits in an HMO plan or to purchase fee-for-service medicine, you occasionally might disagree with a decision that Medicare (or the HMO) has made about your health coverage. Maybe your doctor has billed you more than the agreed-upon fee. Or the program may have ruled that your medical care wasn't covered by Medicare at all.

Errors are sometimes made, usually unintentionally. Fortunately, you can do more than just get angry. There is an appeals process in place that can resolve these disputes. And you should take advantage of the process that can settle these problems.

During an appeal, you may find out that Medicare, in fact, did make an error. Or possibly you misinterpreted the provisions of Part A or B of the program. In either case, the disagreement will be resolved. Even if you end up on the losing end, at least you'll receive a full explanation of why that decision was made.

THE APPEALS PROCESS

When you file an appeal, one or more of the following elements might be involved:

Provider Decisions: In Part A of Medicare, you might receive a notice from the hospital where you were a patient, notifying you that certain services were not covered by Medicare. If you question that judgment, contact the hospital directly, and request an "official Medicare determination." In that case, the hospital can no longer just decide on its own whether a particular service is covered or not; it must file a claim directly with Medicare for a formal ruling. You'll get a letter in the mail—called a Notice of Utilization—that provides the government's decision on the dispute. At that point, if you continue to believe that an error has been made, read the guidelines that appear on the notice, instructing you how to take the appeal to the next step.

If your care under Part A was received at a skilled nursing facility, or if it involved hospice care or home health care, a so-called "Medicare intermediary" will handle the dispute. Once a decision has been made, you are given 60 days to ask for a reconsideration if you wish, making that request either to the intermediary or to the Social Security Administration. After that, if you are still unhappy, you can appeal once more, this time either to an administrative law judge (for amounts involving $100 or more) or to a federal court (if $1000 or *more is involved*).

PROs, or Peer Review Organizations, can also make decisions about your care. These PROs are panels of doctors to whom the federal government assigns the task of reviewing hospital care and policies as they apply to the Medicare system. For example, they can evaluate claims and examine the necessity of particular care and whether it was delivered in the most appropriate place (for instance, a hospital versus a skilled nursing facility). If you receive notice that a PRO has made a decision about your care that you believe is unfair, you can appeal that decision. If the PRO's "reconsideration decision" still goes against you, and the amount in dispute is at least $200, you can request that an administrative law judge hear the case. If $2,000 or more is contested, you can take your appeal directly to a federal court.

For Part B of Medicare, the appeals process works a little differently. If your doctor knows that Medicare will not pay for a particular treatment under Part B coverage, he or she must explain that in writing—and *give you this notice in advance of receiving the treatment*. If he or she has not done so, you can not be held responsible for paying the bill once the care is given.

Sometimes, you may decide that your physician has made an error, and that the services really should be covered by Medicare. In that case, ask your doctor to request an "Official Medicare Determination" from the government. Even the outcome of this Medicare decision can be appealed, however, first to a Medicare carrier, and then to either an administrative law judge or a federal court, depending on the amount of the medical charges involved in the case.

Prepayment Plans: If you get your medical care from an HMO or other type of prepayment program, the plan itself must notify you in writing if particular coverage is being denied. In that notice, you must also be informed of the procedures available to you to appeal that decision, typically within a 60-day period. If you file an appeal to the HMO and it is denied, then you can ask that the government's Health Care Financing Administration make a judgment on the case. Even if the HCFA decision goes against you, there's still another review available to you from either an administrative law judge (in cases involving at least $100) or a federal court (for cases of $1,000 or more).

Although most disputes can be settled without legal assistance, if you seem to be getting the runaround from one bureaucracy or another, contact a lawyer who specializes in this area. Particularly if the disagreement is over a significant amount of money, a legal consultation may be worth the price.

Do You Qualify for Medicaid?

If you are elderly or disabled, and have a low income and limited savings, the Medicaid program in your state may pay your Medicare costs in full, including premiums, deductibles and co-payments. Although states can structure the program in their own ways, including instituting differences in the criteria they use to determine whether an individual qualifies for Medicaid help, here is a general picture of regulations that may apply where you live:

- You must qualify for Part A of Medicare.

- Your yearly income must fall below a certain level. In 1992, that figure was $7,050 for one person, and $9,430 for a family of two.

- Your savings (including bank accounts, stocks and bonds) must not exceed $4,000 per individual, or $6,000 per couple. Certain assets are usually excluded in this calculation of your net worth, such as your home, car, furniture, burial plot and life insurance.

Medicaid also might pay for your Part B coverage. Again, check on the qualifications guidelines in your state. In general, you may be able to participate in this program if your income is less than 110 percent of the federal poverty criteria.

Is Medigap for You?

As we mentioned early in this chapter, Medicare will give you good, basic protection. But it won't take care of everything. Because of the gaps in Medicare, a large private industry has arisen, selling supplemental insurance policies that provide coverage for many services that Medicare does not include.

Until 1991, insurance companies flooded the market with their own carefully crafted and aggressively marketed "Medigap" plans that often confused customers more than they relieved their concerns. But since then, Medigap policies have become standardized by law. That means that insurance companies can offer only up to ten standardized plans (which are identified by the letters A through J)—although some plans are not offered in every state. Plan A is the most basic policy, providing a "core package" of benefits. The remaining plans add various additional benefits to the basic coverage.

To help you evaluate a Medigap plan, ask the insurance agent the following questions—and confirm the agent's answers by reading the policy itself:

• **What coverage does the plan offer beyond Medicare's basic protection?** For instance, are you covered for extra days in the hospital or in a skilled nursing home? Are the costs of outpatient prescription medications paid for? What about private duty nursing? Or custodial care

> *If you are elderly or disabled, and have a low income and limited savings, the Medicaid program in your state may pay your Medicare costs in full, including premiums, deductibles and co-payments.*

(bathing, dressing, feeding) in a nursing home? By re-reading this chapter, you'll get a good sense of what's excluded in Medicare, and what you need to look for in a Medigap policy.

• **Does the plan pay for the deductibles and co-payments that you would be responsible for in Parts A and B?** Remember, the co-payments alone usually leave you obligated to pay 20 percent of covered services. For a major operation that might cost $20,000 or more, your 20 percent portion can become a significant burden. Make sure your supplemental policy picks up these potentially large payments.

• **Does the policy start to cover pre-existing conditions no later than three to six months after the plan goes into force?** Pre-existing conditions are medical problems that you've been treated for in the recent past. If you buy your Medigap policy early (see the explanation of "open enrollment period" below), these exclusion periods are limited to six months—and they are barred completely in Medigap policies that you've bought to replace an existing one, if the original policy had been in force for at least six months. Also, you can often buy a "rider" or additional insurance that will cover you for these medical problems immediately.

• **Is the policy "guaranteed renewable"—that is, even if you develop a serious illness, can you continue to renew your insurance, and not face cancellation by the insurance company?** Although the law now mandates that this clause be part of Medigap coverage, cancellation is still legally possible under two circumstances: if you fail to pay your monthly premiums, or if you knowingly misstated information on your original application.

• **What is the annual cost of the policy?** Of course, the broader your protection, the better. However, keep in mind that the more comprehensive policies also will probably be more costly. Evaluate what you can cover out of your own pocket; if you can realistically afford certain charges, you can obtain a less expensive Medigap policy. For instance, if you can pay the $100 deductible for Part B of Medicare

What Is the Basic Medigap Policy?

In many states, you can choose from as many as ten standardized Medigap policies. The most basic of these plans, called Plan A, offers a "core package" of fundamental benefits. It includes coverage for:

- Your co-insurance in Part A (for hospital days 61 through 90, and for Medicare's 60 lifetime reserve days) and Part B (20 percent of approved charges).

- A maximum of 365 additional days of hospital care under the provisions of Part A, once Medicare's benefits end.

- Three pints of blood each year (Under Part A, you are obligated to pay for the first three pints of blood; under Part B, you must pay your 20 percent co-insurance for the cost of all blood beyond the third pint).

Other policies may add benefits to this basic package, including:

- Your deductibles in Parts A and B.

- The co-payments you must pay for skilled nursing care.

- Excess doctors' fees (beyond the approved charges), typically covering 80 or 100 percent of charges.

- Prescription medications (typically, a 50 percent co-payment after a $250 deductible is met, with a cap of either $1,250 or $3,000).

- Preventive care (up to a maximum of $120 per year).

- Coverage while traveling in foreign countries (Medicare pays for your health care only when it is delivered in the U.S.).

without putting a strain on your finances, buy a policy that doesn't cover it, and reduce your insurance premiums.

A large private industry has arisen, selling supplemental insurance policies that provide coverage for many services that Medicare does not include.

• **What if an insurance agent tries to sell you two Medigap policies, trying to convince you that the more coverage you have, the better?** We suggest looking for another insurance agent. Not only do you need just one policy—why duplicate your benefits and spend more money, too?—but the law *prohibits* an insurer from selling you a second one. If you already have an existing Medigap policy, you must agree to let it lapse in order to purchase a new one.

As with other aspects of Medicare, the earlier you purchase a Medigap policy, the better off you may be. After all, if you delay, you run the risk of developing a medical problem that an insurance company might consider to be a "pre-existing condition." You are also entitled to certain protection if you apply early. For example:

Let's say your Part B coverage of Medicare goes into effect on August 1, 1994. Under federal law, you have six months from that date—or until February 1, 1995—to obtain Medigap coverage in an "open enrollment period," when you'll find the most advantageous rates. During these six months, you cannot be turned away by an insurance company, nor can the rates be increased because of your health. That's the law.

However, if you wait too long, and your open enrollment period passes by, you could be in trouble. You might find that your monthly premiums for this Medigap coverage have gone up. Even worse, you could have the door slammed in your face by insurers who consider you a bad risk; they could refuse to sell you *any* kind of policy, no matter what the cost.

One additional point: If you belong to an HMO, you probably do not need a Medicare supplemental insurance policy. Your Medicare deductibles and co-payments are already covered. As for additional benefits, ask your HMO about them; they may already be offered at no extra cost.

Where to Get More Information

If you belong to an HMO, you probably do not need a Medicare supplemental insurance policy.

Your local Social Security office can provide you with a copy of *The Medicare Handbook*, which offers a comprehensive look at this government program. You can also order this booklet by calling the toll-free Social Security number, 800-772-1213. Or call the Medicare Hotline at 800-638-6833.

For a copy of the *Guide to Health Insurance for People with Medicare*, a publication from the Health Care Financing Administration, contact the Consumer Information Center, Department 70, Pueblo, CO 81009. This booklet provides information on supplemental insurance and how it works.

PREVENTION TIPS
(WAYS YOU CAN SAVE MONEY—AND STAY WELL)

CHAPTER 8

Many people blame their ill health on bad genes or bad luck when, in fact, bad habits are often at fault. Some bad habits are easy to break. One good example is remembering to buckle up every time you get in the car. It takes virtually no time and very little effort, but could save both your pocketbook and your life should you get in an accident. Other bad habits pose a bigger problem. For the veteran smoker, quitting may seem impossible, just as losing weight may appear a pipe dream to those who are overweight.

But everyone must start somewhere, and—before any changes can be made—you first need to identify where the problems lie. Only by recognizing your unhealthy habits for what they are can you go on to adopt healthier ways. On the following pages, we present more than thirty things that you can do (some big and some small) to promote your own good health and save money as a result.

Don't Smoke

Smoking is the leading cause of preventable illness and death in the United States. It is estimated that medical costs due to smoking total some 72 billion dollars. If you smoke, quitting is one of the easiest

> *If you smoke, quitting is one of the easiest ways to cut your medical bills.*

ways to cut your medical bills (not to mention how much you'll save by not buying cigarettes).

Smokers are two to four times more likely to suffer a heart attack than are nonsmokers because smoking promotes atherosclerosis (hardening of the arteries). Blood vessels elsewhere in the body are also affected by smoking: narrowing of the arteries in the legs can cause pain when you walk; blockage of arteries in the head and neck can result in a stroke.

Cancer is another very serious concern for smokers. Most people are aware by now that smoking causes lung cancer. But the chemicals that smoking puts into your bloodstream can cause several other kinds of cancer, as well, including cancer of the bladder, breast and pancreas.

The damage to the lungs doesn't end with cancer. Smoking also causes scarring of lung tissue, which leads to emphysema, a debilitating lung disease found almost exclusively in people who smoke. And smokers are also more susceptible to pneumonia.

Pregnant women who smoke increase their risk for delivering prematurely and having low-birth-weight babies. Children whose parents smoke are more susceptible to middle ear infections, bronchitis, pneumonia and wheezing. Infants may be at greater risk for sudden infant death if their parents smoke.

The list of smoking-related costs goes on and on. Smoking is associated with an increased risk of cataracts, osteoporosis and stomach ulcers. And the relationship between smoking and dental problems should be no great surprise to those who bear the yellow stains characteristic of a smoker's teeth.

But what if you've been smoking for a long time? Does quitting make a difference, or is the damage already done? The answer is absolutely positive. Although it doesn't happen overnight, quitting smoking can reduce your medical risks to nearly those of a person who's never smoked. Ten years after quitting, your risk for heart disease is nearly identical to that of a lifelong nonsmoker and, five years later (fifteen years after kicking the habit), your risk of developing lung cancer is only slightly higher than that of nonsmokers.

Maintain a Smoke-free Environment

It is estimated that between 30,000 and 50,000 people die in the United States each year not because they smoke but because they inhale second-hand smoke produced by people smoking around them. That's a high price to pay for someone else's bad habit.

Even if the serious medical consequences of second-hand smoke don't frighten you, you should be concerned about the more subtle effects it

Lung Cancer Is Only the Tip of the Iceberg

Did you know that smoking also causes cancer of the mouth, throat, stomach and esophagus. Smoking is even a risk factor for cancers of such organs as the pancreas, kidneys and bladder!

The US Surgeon General has estimated that smoking causes:

- 79 percent of all cases of lung cancer in women
  90 percent of all cases of lung cancer in men

- 87 percent of all cases of laryngeal cancer in women
  81 percent of all cases of laryngeal cancer in men

- 61 percent of all cases of oral cancer in women
  92 percent of all cases of oral cancer in men

- 75 percent of all cases of esophageal cancer in women
  78 percent of all cases of esophageal cancer in men

- 34 percent of all cases of pancreatic cancer in women
  29 percent of all cases of pancreatic cancer in men

- 12 percent of all cases of kidney cancer in women
  48 percent of all cases of kidney cancer in men

- 37 percent of all cases of bladder cancer in women
  47 percent of all cases of bladder cancer in men.

will have on your health and on the long-term impact it can have on your wallet. Decrease your exposure to cigarette smoke by doing the following:

- Avoid public places with lots of smokers. In restaurants, ask to sit in the nonsmoking section (even if the wait is a little longer). Avoid restaurants that don't provide this courtesy. Better yet, patronize restaurants that are 100 percent nonsmoking.

- Lobby for laws to ban smoking in public places.

Keep Your Blood Cholesterol Under 200

High blood cholesterol is one of the major risk factors for heart disease (the others being male sex, high blood pressure, smoking, a family history of early onset of heart disease, diabetes, and a low level of HDL cholesterol, the so-called "good cholesterol").

As your blood cholesterol level rises, so does your risk of heart attack. A cholesterol level over 300 makes you four times more likely to suffer a heart attack than if you had a cholesterol level of 200. Even cholesterol levels that were once considered safe (in the low-200 range) are now known to carry an increased risk of dying from heart disease.

Lifetime Medical Expenditures

DIFFERENCES BETWEEN SMOKERS AND NONSMOKERS

	Heavy Smokers (more than 25 per day)	*Moderate Smokers* (less than 25 per day)	*Nonsmokers*
Male:	$40,187	$32,891	$27,276
Female:	$60,347	$48,918	$42,783

Source: National Center for Health Statistics, Vol. 70, No. 1, 1992

You may be able to reduce your cholesterol level dramatically just by making simple changes in your diet. If
your blood cholesterol level is very
high or it won't come down sufficient-
ly with dietary modifications alone,
your doctor may recommend cholesterol-lowering medications. Although

> *You may be able to reduce your cholesterol level dramatically just by making simple changes in your diet.*

some of these medications are fairly expensive, their cost is minimal
compared to the cost of treating chronic heart disease.

Take an Aspirin Every Other Day

The U.S. Preventive Task Force recommends low doses of aspirin (325
mg every other day) for men 40 years or older who have risk factors
for coronary artery disease (high total cholesterol, low HDL cholesterol, diabetes, high blood pressure, family history of early-onset
coronary artery disease), provided there are no medical reasons that
prevent the use of aspirin. These recommendations are based on the
results of a study done at Harvard Medical School, which showed a
47 percent reduction in the incidence of heart attacks in men who
used low doses of aspirin regularly.

Currently, the Task Force does not recommend preventive aspirin use
for men without risk factors for heart disease or for women (although
it may in fact be beneficial to these groups) because of concerns about
aspirin's potential side effects (which include an increased risk of
stomach irritation, gastrointestinal bleeding and stroke due to bleeding in the brain). But if you are over 40 (male or female, with or without risk factors for heart disease), we recommend that you discuss the
pros and cons of aspirin therapy with your physician.

Maintain Your Ideal Body Weight

The risks that excess weight poses to health are much more serious
than many people realize. Obesity has been linked to an increased
risk of cancer of the endometrium, breast and colon (and possibly
also to cancer of the cervix, ovary and prostate). Obesity is also both
directly and indirectly associated with heart disease. It not only

> One study estimated that five to eight percent of the costs of all illnesses are related to the problem of obesity.

increases your risk of heart disease but also contributes to the development of high blood pressure and diabetes. Obesity can also contribute to low back pain.

The medical risks of obesity translate into dramatically increased medical bills. One study estimated that five to eight percent of the costs of all illnesses are related to the problem of obesity. In the United States, the economic costs associated with obesity approach $40 billion a year (and that's a conservative figure).

Exercise Regularly

A study at Stanford University Medical School examined the effects of various lifestyle characteristics on longevity in more than 10,000 men. During the seven-year study, men who started a program of moderate sports activity were 23 percent less likely to die than men who did not exercise.

The more the men exercised, the greater the benefit to their health. Men in this study who walked three to eight miles per week were ten percent less likely to die than those who walked less than three miles per week. Men who walked nine or more miles per week reduced their risk of dying even further; they were 22 percent less likely to die than those walking less than three miles per week.

We recommend a comprehensive exercise plan that includes aerobic training, strength training and flexibility training. Choose exercises that you like and experiment with different types of exercises until you find a fitness plan suited to your tastes and needs.

A number of excellent books are available on exercise, from running to weight lifting. For example, *The Rockport Walking Program* by James M. Rippe, MD, with Ann Ward, PhD, and Karla Dougherty, is an excellent source for information on developing a walking program. Your local library or bookstore can provide you with books on the type of exercise of interest to you.

Get Enough Sleep

More than 20 years ago, researchers in California studied a large group of people to see which lifestyle measures made a difference in life expectancy. To no one's surprise, they discovered that not smoking, avoiding obesity and exercising regularly add years to your life. But they also learned that simply sleeping seven to eight hours every night helps, too. We don't know how sleep increases your lifespan, but some experts think it may have something to do with your body's need to rejuvenate itself from the stress of daily living. Others point to the increased accident rate experienced by people who are chronically fatigued. Whatever the reason, getting seven to eight hours of sleep every night is one easy way to enhance your health and reduce your medical bills.

Limit Your Alcohol Consumption

Physical problems related to the use of alcohol range from liver disease to infertility, and cost the nation an estimated $7 billion a year in medical expenses alone. The total cost of alcohol abuse, including lost productivity, premature death, accidents and crime, add up to approximately $85 billion annually.

The life-threatening complications of alcohol abuse include cirrhosis (a serious form of liver disease), pancreatitis (inflammation of the pancreas), and cancer of the mouth and esophagus. Recent evidence suggests that alcohol plays a role in the development of breast cancer. Alcohol intoxication also puts you at increased risk for accidents such as car crashes, drowning, burns and serious falls.

Never Drink and Drive

More than half of all fatalities from car accidents involve alcohol, and not all of them involve "drunk drivers." Just one cocktail puts you in danger by dulling your senses, slowing your reaction time and increasing your chances of falling asleep behind the wheel. And don't ever ride as a passenger in a car with a driver who's been drinking. It's nearly as dangerous as driving under the influence of alcohol yourself.

Don't Drink if You're Pregnant

Drinking during pregnancy places your unborn baby at risk for fetal alcohol syndrome (a group of congenital abnormalities associated with alcohol exposure during pregnancy). No safe level of alcohol has been established during pregnancy and research suggests that even small amounts of alcohol can cause problems for the fetus. We recommend that alcohol be avoided entirely during pregnancy.

Avoid Sun Exposure

While very small amounts of sunshine can be good for you (sun exposure stimulates your skin to manufacture vitamin D), too much sun increases your risk of skin cancer. The greater the exposure, the higher your risk.

Your face and neck are at especially high risk because they are exposed to the sun on a daily basis, while the rest of your body is usually protected by clothing. Here are a few simple rules to cut your risk of skin cancer:

- Wear a hat when outside for any period of time. Hats with a back flap can help protect your neck.
- When you're outside, always use a sunscreen with a sun protection factor of 15 (SPF-15) on exposed parts of your body. Less protective sunscreens may allow you to burn if the sun is strong or your exposure is prolonged. Reapply sunscreen frequently. Women who use cosmetics should choose brands that include sunscreen.

Eat Smart

EAT MORE FRUITS AND VEGETABLES

Your parents always told you to "Eat your vegetables." Well, they were right. Several recent studies have shown that the consumption of fruits and vegetables is linked to a reduction in the occurrence of cancer. Other studies show that diets high in fruits and vegetables increase your life expectancy.

Fruits and vegetables are some of the best sources of vitamins and minerals. An orange contains 66 mg of vitamin C—more than 100 percent of the RDA; a carrot contains over 7,000 IUs of vitamin A, more than 100 percent of the RDA; and 2/3 cup of broccoli contains about 200 mcg of vitamin K, more than 100 percent of the RDA.

INCLUDE PLENTY OF FIBER IN YOUR DIET

While dietary fiber contains no calories, it is another important part of a healthy diet. People who eat little fiber appear to be at higher risk for some forms of cancer. By speeding up the passage of stool through the colon, fiber decreases the time the colon is exposed to potentially dangerous waste products and so may reduce your risk of colon cancer. By producing soft stools that move quickly through the colon, fiber also helps prevent constipation.

High-fiber diets also may reduce your risk of heart disease by helping to lower your blood cholesterol levels. Fiber does this by preventing the body's absorption of substances that could be used by the liver to manufacture cholesterol.

The easiest and best way to get the fiber you need is by eating fruits, vegetables and whole-grain cereals and breads. If you can't get enough fiber this way, fiber supplements may help.

LIMIT YOUR INTAKE OF ALL FATS

A low-fat diet can decrease your medical risks—and costs—in several ways:

- It helps you control your weight. Foods high in fat are dense in calories. One gram of fat has more than twice the number of calories as the same amount of either protein or carbohydrate—9 calories per gram compared to 4 calories per gram. That means if you stay away from foods high in fat you can eat larger quantities of food without taking in as many calories, so you can actually eat more without gaining weight.

- A low-fat diet helps lower your cholesterol level. Fats, particularly saturated fats, are converted into cholesterol by your body. By lowering the fat content of your diet, you can lower your blood cholesterol level and decrease your risk of developing heart disease.

- Decreasing the amount of fat you eat can also help lower your risk of developing some cancers (particularly of the colon and breast). Fat intake should be limited to no more than 30 percent of your total caloric intake and, in general, the less fat you eat the better (except for children under two, who should not be on a fat-restricted diet). For example, if you consume 2100 calories a day, fewer than 700 calories should be from fats.

REDUCE YOUR INTAKE OF SATURATED FATS

All fats are not created equal. While they are all high in calories (9 calories per gram), saturated fat is worse for your heart than others. If you have high or borderline high blood cholesterol levels, it's especially important to decrease your intake of saturated fats.

Chemically, the difference between saturated and unsaturated fats is the number of hydrogen atoms they contain (saturated fats contain more than unsaturated fats). Medically, the difference is far more dramatic. Saturated fats are easily converted into cholesterol by your body (in fact, saturated fats can cause your blood cholesterol levels to rise even more than dietary cholesterol itself).

Saturated fats remain solid at room temperature. Two examples of saturated fats are butter and shortening. By cutting saturated fats out of your diet, you reduce your body's ability to manufacture cholesterol and lower your risk of developing heart disease. The National Cholesterol Education Program (NCEP) recommends that less than ten percent of your daily calories come from saturated fat; that compares with the 15 to 20 percent presently consumed by the average American.

SUPPLEMENT YOUR DIET WITH SELECTED VITAMINS AND MINERALS

Until recently, there wasn't enough scientific evidence to suggest that taking supplements really made a difference in your health. However, recent research has clearly demonstrated that high levels of selected vitamins can produce dramatic health benefits—including reducing your risk of heart disease, certain cancers and cataracts.

Several studies have shown that the so-called "antioxidant" vitamins (vitamins A, C and E) and selenium may reduce your risk of several chronic diseases and actually help battle the aging process. They appear to accomplish this by destroying substances known as free radicals, dangerous particles that are the byproduct of the body's normal metabolism. Free radicals cause injury to cells and appear to play a role in the development of numerous diseases, including cancer, heart disease and cataracts.

While it is possible for many people to get the vitamins and minerals they need from their diet, it is difficult to get enough of the antioxidant vitamins. The reality is that most of us simply don't eat well enough every day to ensure adequate nutrition. We eat on the run, we eat out, we skip meals, we go on diets—for whatever reason, we don't consume the amounts of vitamins and minerals that the new studies suggest we need.

Some people—no matter how hard they try—are probably not able to meet their needs through diet. This group includes babies and older people, who consume very small quantities of food; people who are chronically ill; people who are on diets; and women who are pregnant or about to get pregnant. For these people, dietary supplements are a must. We'd like to call your attention to the following nutrients in particular.

CALCIUM (1200 MG CALCIUM)   Calcium is an essential mineral for bones, neuromuscular activity and the regulation of blood pressure.

Osteoporosis, a condition in which bones begin to lose calcium—and so become more brittle and prone to fracture—presents an enormous health problem (and, therefore, a major financial problem), principally to postmenopausal women. About 15 percent of all women suffer a hip fracture during their lifetime, costing the nation an estimated $7 billion annually.

Because the risks associated with calcium supplementation are minimal, we advocate that men and women of all ages maintain a daily calcium intake of 1200 mg. If you have kidney stones, you should discuss the use of calcium supplements with your physician before using them.

VITAMIN C (250 MG)   Vitamin C, touted as a cure for everything from cancer to the common cold, is beginning to live up to at least part of its reputation. Recent studies suggest that vitamin C does have the ability to prevent certain chronic diseases and at the least helps battle symptoms of the common cold.

> *Vitamin C, touted as a cure for everything from cancer to the common cold, is beginning to live up to at least part of its reputation.*

The research shows that vitamin C may play a role in the prevention of several cancers, including breast, colon, mouth, stomach, lung, cervix and prostate. And a study performed at the University of California, Los Angeles, suggests that heart disease can be prevented (and life prolonged) with vitamin C supplementation. Men and women who supplemented their diets with 250 mg of vitamin C each day were found to lower their risk of heart disease and live significantly longer than those who did not (one year longer for women and up to five years for men).

Vitamin C—alone or in combination with vitamin E—may also play an important role in reducing your risk of cataracts. In one study, people taking 300 to 500 mg of vitamin C and 400 IU of vitamin E reduced their risk of developing cataracts by more than 50 percent.

The current RDA for vitamin C is 60 mg/day. We recommend using supplemental vitamin C to bring your daily intake up to 250 mg. The risks associated with vitamin C supplements at this level are minimal and are significantly outweighed by the potential benefits.

VITAMIN E (100 IU)   For years people have been using vitamin E to treat nearly every ailment imaginable, from sunburns and stretch marks to heart disease and wrinkles. Most of this use has been subjected to heavy criticism from the general medical community.

However, recent studies support a role for vitamin E in the battle against several chronic diseases. A study conducted by researchers at Harvard Medical School found that men and women who supplemented their diet with at least 100 units of vitamin E per day for at least two and a half years had up to 40 percent fewer heart attacks than a similar group who did not use supplements (or who used lower doses). Vitamin E also appears to play a role in the prevention of some forms of cancer and in the prevention of cataracts. We recommend a supplemental dose of 100 IU of vitamin E per day. This dose surpasses the US RDA requirement of 30 IU per day. We suggest the higher dose as most studies indicate that it is necessary to achieve significant benefit. Also, at the 100 IU dosage, toxicity risk is minimal and we believe benefits outweigh risks.

BETA CAROTENE Traditionally, beta carotene has been considered little more than a good source of vitamin A (beta carotene is converted into vitamin A by the body), but recent evidence suggests that its abilities as an antioxidant are at least as important. The role of beta carotene in the prevention of several types of cancer is now well documented and preliminary studies from Harvard suggest that beta carotene may also significantly reduce your risk of developing heart disease.

In and of itself, beta carotene is not considered an essential nutrient, provided your diet contains a sufficient amount of other sources of vitamin A. However, we recommend that you use beta carotene as a primary way to fulfill your daily vitamin A requirements. In that way, you not only satisfy your body's needs for vitamin A but you also benefit from beta carotene's antioxidant capabilities. As vitamin A is stored in the liver, it can build up to toxic levels. The effects of this toxicity include elevated pressure in the brain, headaches, blurred vision, dermatitis and hair loss. Beta carotene, unlike vitamin A, is *not* stored in the body and so is not a risk for reaching toxic levels.

FOLIC ACID Several studies have shown that supplementation of the diet with folic acid before conception and during pregnancy can reduce a woman's risk of bearing a child with congenital deformities of the spinal cord and brain (spina bifida and anencephaly, also called neural tube defects). These devastating developmental abnormalities occur with surprising frequency, affecting nearly 4,000 babies per year in the United States. For women who have had one infant with a neural tube defect, the risk of giving birth to another child with this problem is even higher in subsequent pregnancies.

In one study reported in *The New England Journal of Medicine*, there were no cases of neural tube defects among 2104 women taking multivitamin supplements that included 800 micrograms of folic acid per day for several months before and after conception and six cases among 1052 women who did not receive the supplements.

We recommend that all women of childbearing age supplement their diets with 400 micrograms per day of folic acid.

Always Wear Your Safety Belt

Several million people are injured each year in car accidents, nearly half of them requiring some form of medical treatment. Nearly 50,000 Americans die each year in motor vehicle accidents. Safety belts, if worn regularly by everyone, could reduce these numbers by half.

Wearing a safety belt not only protects your health, it spares your checkbook. A study by University of Chicago researchers compared injuries and hospital charges that safety belt and non-safety belt wearers incurred as a result of car accidents. People who wore safety belts suffered injuries that were significantly less severe and required admission to the hospital almost 65 percent less often. What kind of savings did this generate? Hospital charges were 66 percent lower for people who wore their safety belts ($534 compared to $1583).

Always Use Approved Child Safety Seats

Car seats are required by law in all fifty states. Unfortunately, recent studies show that many parents are not using them properly, or not using the seat at all on short trips (a potentially deadly mistake). Every year, car crashes are the cause of more deaths in children between the ages of one and fourteen than any other reason, medical or otherwise.

Many of these deaths could be prevented if the children were properly restrained. One study showed that children in restraint devices are almost three times more likely to escape from a car accident uninjured than are children not using restraints, while the injuries they did suffer were much less severe. If you ever take your child in a car, the single most important thing you can do for your child is to buy, properly install, and routinely use a federally approved car seat.

Contrary to what many people believe, a parent's lap is actually the most dangerous place for a child to ride. In case of a crash, you probably wouldn't be able to hold on to your child. But even if you could, your body would crush the child if you were thrown against the dashboard yourself.

Here are some guidelines to help you select, install and use a car seat.

> *Children in restraint devices are almost three times more likely to escape from a car accident uninjured than are children not using restraints.*

- All new car seats today must meet federal safety guidelines. Don't use a seat made before 1982, the year these regulations went into effect. For a list of acceptable seats that are available today, ask your pediatrician or write to the American Academy of Pediatrics, Shopping Guide, 141 Northwest Point Road, P.O. Box 927, Elk Grove Village, Illinois 60009.

- The most effective restraint is a five-point harness that consists of two shoulder straps, a lap belt and a crotch strap. A padded armrest in front of your child may be more comfortable, but it does not provide extra protection and is not a substitute for a harness.

- The center of the back seat is the safest place for a seat to be installed. To provide maximum protection for your child, it is essential that the seat be installed correctly, so follow the manufacturer's installation instructions precisely.

- Choose a car seat that is convenient to use. You're more likely to use it if it's easier to get your child in and out.

Always Wear a Bicycle Helmet

Each year there are more than a half-million emergency room visits and over 1000 deaths resulting from biking accidents. Head injuries are the leading cause of death from these accidents. Yet, despite the fact that bicycle helmets have been shown to reduce the risk of head injury by as much as 85 percent, less than ten percent of bicyclists wear helmets. Be sure to wear a helmet every time you ride a bike.

Install Smoke Detectors and Fire Alarms

If a fire occurs, the earlier you discover it, the greater your chance of putting it out or escaping from it. Today, your best tools for an early warning are smoke detectors; they can reduce your risk of dying in a fire by up to 50 percent.

Install smoke detectors throughout your home, mounting them on the ceiling or on the wall 6 to 12 inches from the ceiling. Place them in halls just outside bedrooms, in the living room, garage and other areas where they can detect smoke as it approaches the bedrooms.

Remember that fire and smoke alarms are only effective if they're working. As many as one-third of installed alarms are thought to be inoperable, usually because their batteries are dead. You should check your alarms monthly to be sure they are working properly, and replace your batteries at least once a year.

Turn Down Your Water Heater (to 120 Degrees Fahrenheit)

Hundreds of millions of dollars a year are spent treating burns, a large number of which are scald burns. This type of burn is excruciatingly painful and can cause permanent scarring and deformity.

Scald burns are most frequently caused by setting the hot water thermostat too high or by spilling hot cooking liquids on the skin. By turning down your central water heater, you can reduce the danger of an accidental burn in the tub or shower. This is especially important if you have a young child at home who is able to turn a bathtub faucet or an older person who could fall in the shower with the hot water running. Set your thermostat to no more than 120 degrees Fahrenheit (48 degrees Celsius). Anti-scald devices are also available and can be attached to most faucets. These will automatically turn off the water if the temperature rises too high.

Practice Water Safety

Did you know that drowning is the third-most common cause of death in children under the age of five? Most of these drownings occur in swimming pools. Pools without some form of barrier around them are particularly dangerous. The best way to prevent children from getting into trouble in a swimming pool is to keep them from getting near it in the first place. Pool fencing has been shown to reduce the risk of drownings and near drownings by up to 90 percent.

> *The best way to prevent children from getting into trouble in a swimming pool is to keep them from getting near it in the first place.*

Although swimming classes for young children are widely available, the American Academy of Pediatrics does not recommend them for children under the age of three for the following reasons:

- You may be lulled into being less cautious because you think your child can swim.

- Young children who are repeatedly immersed in water may tend to swallow large amounts. This can lead to a problem known as water intoxication, which can result in convulsions, shock, and even death.

When your child reaches three, you may want to consider swimming lessons, but remember that even a child who knows how to swim needs to be watched constantly. Young children can drown in only a few inches of water, so never leave a young child alone near water, not even for a moment.

Here are a few more water safety guidelines you should always keep in mind:

- Children who are swimming, even in a shallow toddler's pool, should be watched by an adult, preferably one who knows cardio-pulmonary resuscitation (CPR).

- Enforce general safety rules: no running near the pool; no pushing others underwater; and no diving into the shallow end.

- Don't allow children to use inflatable toys or mattresses to keep them afloat. These toys may deflate suddenly, or the child may slip off.

- Keep a safety ring with a rope beside the pool at all times.

Prevent Falls

PREVENTING FALLS IN CHILDREN

Falls are an almost inescapable part of childhood, but there are many things you can do to keep your child from being seriously injured as a result of a fall.

- Install gates at the top and bottom of stairs. Hold on to the banister yourself with one hand whenever you are going up or down the stairs while carrying your child.

- Open windows from the top, if possible. If you must open them from the bottom, install window bars or screens that only an adult or older child can push out from the inside. Never put chairs, sofas or low tables (or anything else a child might climb on) in front of a window.

- Never leave your child alone on high places—not even for a second.

PREVENTING FALLS IN ADULTS

Accidental falls are a very common cause of injuries at any age, but the problem increases dramatically as people age and their muscles lose strength and their bones become more brittle. The loss of strength makes it much more difficult for them to "catch" themselves, while brittle bones increase the likelihood of fractures and other serious injuries.

Among older people living at home, about one-third will experience a fall in a given year. Among older people living in an institution, about two-thirds will have a fall in the same period of time. Of all those who fall, about five percent will be seriously injured. Among people 65 or older, falls are responsible for about eight percent of all hospitalizations. They are the number-one cause for nursing home placement and the fifth leading cause of death. Needless to say, these injuries lead to astronomical medical costs, not all of which are covered by Medicare.

Nearly two-thirds of the falls at home could be prevented by removing physical hazards or making simple modifications to the environment. No matter what the age of the people in your household, go through the house and do the following:

- Attach all rugs and carpets securely to the floor at their edges so it is impossible to trip on a loose edge. If you use "throw" rugs, buy only those with a nonslip backing or nail the rugs to the floor.

- Eliminate all electrical cords and telephone cords that cross traffic paths.

- Install handrails in bathtubs, showers, and all other locations where a person may need some support.

- Put adhesive bath mats in tubs and showers.

- Make sure that all stepstools have handrails and rest solidly on their legs.

- Make sure all traffic areas are brightly lit.

Medications are another significant cause of falls, especially in the elderly. Many medications cause subtle changes in coordination and strength; others can make you dizzy or drowsy. Side effects can sometimes become overwhelming in the elderly, when slight changes in strength, coordination or gait can be enough to cause a fall. If you are having symptoms, review your medications and their potential side effects with your doctor. Your doctor may be able to switch you to another medication with fewer side effects or lower the dose of the medication you are currently taking.

Prevent Poisonings

Each year, about 100,000 children are victims of poisoning. Ninety percent of these children are under the age of five. It's natural for children that young to be curious, and that curiosity leads them to reach for anything they can get their hands on. Unfortunately, what they get their hands on tends to end up in the mouth.

Here are some ways to reduce the likelihood that your child will be a poisoning victim:

- Use cabinet slide locks and latches to lock medications and other hazardous substances in your medicine cabinet.

- Buy and keep medications in containers with child-proof caps.

- Throw away prescription medicines when the illness for which they were prescribed has passed.

- Store hazardous products in their original containers in locked cabinets that are out of your child's reach. Do not keep detergents and other cleaning products under the sink unless they are in a cabinet with a safety lock.

- If your child ingests any substance that may be poisonous, call your local Poison Control Center immediately. Post the Poison Control's number near every telephone in your home, along with other emergency numbers.

Say No to Drugs

Millions of Americans indulge in a variety of illicit substances such as marijuana, cocaine and heroine, with seemingly little regard for the devastating effects these drugs can have. The economic consequences are staggering, the medical consequences alone amounting to billions and billions of dollars.

The recent deaths of several of the country's finest athletes have awakened the nation to the dangers of cocaine. Cocaine use can induce heart attacks, even in the most well-conditioned heart, as well as cause bleeding in the brain and seizures. Perhaps the most distressing effects of cocaine are those experienced by infants born to mothers who used cocaine while they were pregnant. To understand the effects of cocaine on the unborn fetus, one need only look at neonatal intensive care units across the country—where premature infants are struggling to survive (needless to say, at a very high human and economic cost).

For every 1000 heroin addicts, 10 die each year as a result of their habit. But you don't have to be a regular user to put yourself at risk. If used intravenously, after just one experience with heroin, you could find yourself infected with the virus that causes AIDS.

The use of drugs by adolescents and young adults is perhaps the saddest part of the problem. Nowadays, the pressure to "do" drugs is enormous and children have to be taught ways to resist pressure from peers gracefully. Education and example are the best defense.

Practice Safe Sex (and Educate Your Children About Safe Sex)

Sexually transmitted diseases (STDs) are on the upswing. Several million cases of chlamydia and gonorrhea are diagnosed every year in the United States and hundreds of thousands of new infections with the herpes virus are seen. In addition, syphilis, which had been temporarily brought under control, has been increasing steadily in recent years.

While antibiotics have made many STDs treatable, when left untreated many of these conditions can lead to serious complications. Pelvic inflammatory disease, a complication of chlamydial and gonorrheal infection, can cause infertility in women, while syphilis can lead to irreversible and severe neurological problems. For other conditions, such as hepatitis B and AIDS, there really is no universally effective treatment and the consequences can be deadly.

Infections are not the only potential complication of unprotected intercourse. Without adequate birth control, pregnancy can, and often does, result. Despite the variety of birth control options available, it's thought that nearly 40 percent of all pregnancies among women aged 15 to 44 are unintended.

Although abstaining from sex is the best way to prevent both sexually transmitted diseases and unintended pregnancy, it is not always practical. If you are not in a mutually monogamous sexual relationship, condoms (along with a spermicide containing nonoxynol 9) should always be used to minimize your risk of pregnancy and infection. Because condom use does not completely protect you against pregnancy and infection, the U.S. Preventive Services Task Force recommends that condoms be used in accordance with the following guidelines for condom use:

- Latex condoms, rather than natural membrane condoms, should be used. Torn condoms, those in damaged packages, or those showing signs of age (brittle, sticky, discolored) should not be used.

- The condom should be put on an erect penis, before any intimate contact, and should be unrolled completely to the base.

- A space should be left at the tip of the condom to collect semen; air pockets in the space should be removed by pressing the air out toward the base.

- Water-based lubricants should be used. Those made with petroleum jelly, mineral oil, cold cream, and other oil-based lubricants should not be applied because they may damage the condom.

- Insertion of nonoxynol 9 in the condom increases protection, but vaginal application in addition to condom use is likely to provide greater protection.

- If a condom breaks, it should be replaced immediately.

- After ejaculation and while the penis is still erect, the penis should be withdrawn while carefully holding the condom against the base of the penis so that the condom remains in place.

- Condoms should never be reused.

Although many people would like to deny that their children are sexually active, sex has become a way of life for many teenagers. And teens don't appear to be taking the needed precautions; rates of teenage pregnancy have skyrocketed in recent years as have the number of cases of sexually transmitted diseases among adolescents.

Contrary to the notion that talking about sex will cause your children to become sexually active, discussing sex openly with your children at a very young age is probably the biggest favor you can do them. Your children will learn about sex whether you want them to or not. It's up to you to make sure they get the best information.

Say No to Guns

The misuse of firearms is a significant cause of injuries in the home. Tragically, many of these injuries occur when people are cleaning or playing with a gun they thought was unloaded. In 1990, handguns were responsible for an estimated 800 home accident fatalities.

Children are at particularly high risk of accidental injury. They are naturally curious and have no sense of the dangers involved. If they see a gun, chances are they'll think it's a toy and play with it. That can be deadly. Each year more than 100 children under the age of five are killed by firearms.

The best way to decrease the risk of an accidental shooting in your home is to keep guns out of the house altogether. If you must keep a gun, follow these precautions:

- Take the National Rifle Association's home firearm safety course.

- Always store guns unloaded and in a locked cabinet, far out of the reach of children.

- Lock up all ammunition in a secure and separate location from the firearms.

Perform Regular Self-Examinations

Self-examinations can play an important part in the early detection and diagnosis of cancer. No one knows your body as well as you do. By examining your body at regular intervals, you can pick up potential problems at an early stage, while they are more curable at less cost.

DO REGULAR BREAST SELF-EXAMINATION (MEN, TOO) Breast self-examination should be done once a month. Be on the alert for lumps; nipple discharge; dimpling or discoloration of the skin; or distortion, scaliness or tenderness of the nipple. Your gynecologist or primary care doctor can teach you how to perform a self-exam properly.

EXAMINE YOUR TESTICLES REGULARLY Testicular cancer strikes about 5,000 American men a year. Although it accounts for only one percent

> *All skin cancers are curable if diagnosed and removed early enough.*

of all cancers in men, it is the most common cancer among men between the ages of 15 and 40. Testicular cancer is one of the most curable of all cancers, with cure rates of up to 95 percent if it is found in its earliest stages.

The key to early diagnosis is testicular self-exam. Every man between the ages of 15 and 40 should do a self-exam at least once a month. Start by standing in front of a mirror and looking for any swelling in the skin of the scrotum. Using both hands, examine each testicle by placing the index and middle fingers under the testicle while the thumbs are placed on top. Then gently roll the testicle between the thumbs and the fingers. During the exam, you will also feel the epididymis, a soft, tubelike structure at the back of the testicle.

It is normal for one testicle to be a little larger than the other, but you should call your doctor immediately if you find any unusual swelling, lump or area of unusual firmness. If you have any questions about how to perform this examination properly, ask your personal physician to show you how.

DO REGULAR SELF-EXAMINATIONS OF YOUR SKIN   The most common cancer in both men and women is skin cancer. Though some types of skin cancer are unlikely to spread elsewhere in the body, others can spread widely and even lead to death. Essentially, all skin cancers are curable if diagnosed and removed early enough, so self-examination of the skin is an important tool. At least once every 90 days, with the help of a mirror (or a friend), you should examine every square inch of your body (even the soles of your feet). Pay particular attention to any mole or sore on the skin, and look for the following:

- Changes in size, shape, color, thickness or texture.
- Crusting, bleeding or scabbing that fails to heal or heals and then opens up again.
- Sores or growths that itch, peel or hurt.
- New skin growths.
- Irregular borders or borders that change. If any of these signs appear, see your primary care physician or a dermatologist (skin specialist) without delay.

Keep Up-to-Date with Immunizations

Immunizations are one of the simplest ways you can protect your child. They prevent several serious diseases that have disabling, even life-threatening, consequences. These include hepatitis, diphtheria, and polio, among others.

If every child in the United States was immunized and you didn't travel anywhere outside the country with your child, we might not feel as strongly about immunizing a particular child, since that child's chance of catching an infectious disease would be next to nothing. But, unfortunately, this isn't the reality. Immunization levels are currently dangerously low in the United States, in part because so many parents have neglected to immunize their children and partly because many children have immigrated to the United States in recent years who were not adequately immunized. These conditions make it possible for widespread epidemics to occur. For this reason, we strongly advocate immunizing every child unless there is a medical reason not to do so.

Childhood immunization is an ongoing process, not a "one-shot deal." The first immunizations are generally given shortly after your child is born and they continue well into the child's teens. The American Academy of Pediatrics recommends the immunization schedule shown on the next page for all healthy children. (For children with special health problems, this regimen may require modification.) The following vaccinations are recommended:

DTP (Diphtheria and tetanus toxoids and pertussis vaccine) For the fourth and fifth doses of diphtheria-tetanus pertussis (those given at 15 to 18 months and 4 to 6 years), the acellular (DTaP) can be substituted for the DTP vaccine.

OPV (ORAL POLIO VACCINE) Children in close contact with people with AIDS or on immunosuppressive medications should receive inactivated polio vaccine.

MMR (MEASLES, MUMPS AND RUBELLA VACCINE) If measles is a problem where you live, the schedule for MMR may differ. Contact your local health department for more information.

IMMUNIZATION SCHEDULE

AGE	DTP	OPV	MMR	HBV	Hib	Td
Birth				√		
1–2 months				√		
2 months	√	√			√	
4 months	√	√			√	
6 months	√				√	
6–18 months				√		
12–15 months					√	
15 months			√			
15–18 months	√	√				
4–6 years	√	√				
11–12 years			√	√		
14–16 years				√		√

Source: The American Academy of Pediatrics

HBV (HEPATITIS B VACCINE)   The vaccination schedule may vary depending on the mother's hepatitis B status.

Hib (HAEMOPHILUS INFLUENZA TYPE B)   Hib is a virus which can cause meningitis, pneumonia and infections of the blood, joints, bones, soft tissues, throat and the covering of the heart. There are several different vaccines available—HibTITER and PedvaxHIB. The vaccine selected initially determines the precise immunization schedule and should be used for the full course of immunization.

Td (TETANUS-DIPHTHERIA VACCINE).   This vaccine does not include the pertussis vaccine.

REMEMBER THAT ADULTS NEED IMMUNIZATIONS, TOO

Too many people think that immunizations are only for children. In fact, adults (and the elderly in particular) need immunizations, too. As is the case with children, adult immunizations save millions of dollars and much pain and suffering.

> *Immunizations are one of the simplest ways you can protect your child.*

As you get older, your immune system, your body's natural protection against infection, begins to "lose steam." As a result, you become more susceptible to infections. Immunizations boost your natural immunity and help your body fight off certain infectious illnesses. The U.S. Preventive Service Task Force makes the following recommendations for adults.

PNEUMOCOCCAL VACCINE   All men and women 65 years of age and over should be vaccinated at least once.

The following groups of individuals under 65 years of age should also be immunized:

- Those whose medical conditions place them at high risk of pneumococcal infection, including chronic heart or lung disease, sickle cell anemia, diabetes, severe kidney or liver disease, conditions associated with poor immune function;

- Alcoholics;

- Individuals taking immunosuppressive medications;

- People who have had their spleens removed.

INFLUENZA VACCINE   Individuals 65 years or older should be vaccinated annually.

Before the age of 65, influenza vaccine should be administered to individuals who:

- Reside in chronic care facilities (e.g., nursing homes);

- Have medical conditions such as heart or lung disease, diabetes, kidney disease, and immunosuppressive illnesses that put them at risk of infection ;

- Take immunosuppressive medications;

- Provide health care to a population at high risk for influenza (e.g., doctors, nurses).

HEPATITIS A   Individuals at risk of exposure to hepatitis A require immunization, including:

- Close household and sexual contacts with individuals who have hepatitis A;

- Staff and children at day-care centers and staff and patients of custodial institutions where hepatitis A is occurring;

- Co-workers of food handlers with hepatitis A.

HEPATITIS B   Adults of any age deemed to be at high risk of infection require immunization, including:

- Homosexual men;

- Intravenous drug users;

- People with frequent occupational exposure to blood or blood products (e.g., doctors, nurses, laboratory personnel);

- Following an exposure incident to blood known or suspected to be infected with hepatitis B.

- Susceptible individuals after sexual exposure to an individual infected with hepatitis B.

TETANUS-DIPHTHERIA TOXOID   Adults of any age should be reimmunized at least once every ten years.

MEASLES   All persons born after 1956 who lack evidence of measles immunity (no record that they received live vaccine on or after their first birthday, no laboratory evidence of immunity, and no history of measles infection) should be immunized.

RUBELLA   Susceptible nonpregnant women of childbearing age (no proof of vaccination on or after their first birthday or laboratory evidence of immunity) who agree not to become pregnant for three months should be immunized.

Susceptible pregnant women should be immunized following child-birth.

MUMPS   Susceptible men and women of any age should be immunized.

Take Care of Your Teeth

When most people think of the dentist, they conjure up images of dental drills, major discomfort and big bills. This is an accurate picture for people who neglect their teeth and gums.

More than $34 billion is spent annually on dental services in the United States, most of it for filling cavities, performing root canals and fitting dentures—problems that could have been avoided with proper preventive care.

Here are a few simple steps you should follow to care for your teeth properly and minimize your dental expenses:

BRUSH WELL AT LEAST TWICE A DAY   Brushing does two good things for your teeth. First, it removes plaque, an invisible layer of bacteria that coats your teeth and causes tooth decay. Second, if you use a toothpaste containing fluoride, it exposes your teeth to this cavity-fighting substance. If possible, brush after every meal.

USE TOOTHPASTE WITH FLUORIDE   Fluoride fights cavities by actually combining with tooth enamel to make your teeth stronger and more resistant to decay.

FLOSS BETWEEN TEETH   Flossing removes plaque between teeth that regular brushing can't reach.

LIMIT SNACKS BETWEEN MEALS   The sugar in food reacts with plaque on your teeth and produces acid that can cause tooth decay. Repeated exposure to acid from frequent snacking can result in cavities.

GET REGULAR DENTAL CHECKUPS   Don't wait until you've got a problem to go to the dentist. Regular preventive visits and teeth cleanings will help keep your teeth healthy and allow you to detect problems such as cavities early, when they're less painful and less expensive to treat. The American Dental Association recommends checkups twice a year for most people, although more frequent visits may be necessary for individuals with particular dental problems.

SCREENING

Screening is a way to identify medical problems in their very earliest stages, at a time when they are most easily treated, and when it is most likely that serious problems can be prevented. For example: Routine Pap smears enable physicians to detect and treat abnormalities on the cervix before cervical cancer develops, and blood cholesterol tests can help identify people at high risk for coronary heart disease, most of whom can reduce their risk by making simple dietary changes. Another form of screening is a routine physical exam. Even though you may feel perfectly healthy, the exam gives your doctor an opportunity to find problems before they cause any symptoms.

The idea of regular screening first got a big lift in 1922, when the AMA proposed the concept of annual physical examinations—even for people who were healthy. The idea caught on quickly and gradually expanded over the next few decades to include other kinds of screening procedures, including blood tests, urine tests and chest x-rays. Special laboratories and businesses sprang up just to promote screening, some offering to perform 24 tests or more on a single specimen of blood. It wasn't long before some doctors were ordering these tests on all of their patients at every visit. It was certainly good for business, but how good was it for the patients? The answer: Not good for their health, and especially not good for their pocketbooks.

The truth is, when it comes to screening, you *can* get too much of a good thing. There are direct risks associated with some screening

> The best approach to screening (as with almost everything else in health care) is to balance the potential risks against the potential benefits.

tests: These risks range from painful bruising resulting from a needlestick to an increased rate of cancer from excessive chest or dental x-rays. And there are the risks and costs related to inaccurate screening tests. No test is perfect, so for every thousand tests performed, you've got to assume that some will incorrectly come out negative (meaning they will fail to diagnose a problem that is present), and some will incorrectly come out positive (meaning they will diagnose a problem that doesn't exist). In the first case, you won't be any more at risk than if you hadn't had the screening test (although the test result might give you a false sense of security that leads you to ignore symptoms that show up later). But the latter case—what doctors refer to as a "false positive" result, can start you down an expensive and risky path of further testing. A false positive Pap test report may lead to a biopsy of the cervix, and a false positive test for blood in the stool may lead to telescopic and x-ray examinations of your colon. These procedures are not justified when they are triggered by an inaccurate screening test.

Another problem with some screening tests is that—even though they do detect some problems earlier—they don't always change the final outcome. One example of this is the use of routine pelvic ultrasound tests to screen women for ovarian cancer. The cure rates are no higher for women whose cancers are found this way than for women whose cancers are found during routine pelvic exams. Another example of this problem involves the use of chest x-rays to screen for lung cancer. By the time a lesion is large enough to appear on an x-ray, it's too large to be treated any more effectively than a cancer that's detected after symptoms (usually a cough) arise. So, screening the entire population with chest x-rays doesn't increase the cure rate for those who develop lung cancer, but it does expose everyone else to cancer-causing radiation without offering them any benefit in return.

The best approach to screening (as with almost everything else in health care) is to balance the potential risks against the potential benefits. When a screening test offers a good chance of detecting a problem early enough to make a difference in the way you will be treated or in the outcome of that treatment, and when the test has a high degree of accuracy and a low level of associated risks and cost, it makes sense to get it. When the opposite is true, you are wasting your money and exposing yourself to unnecessary risk.

For example, if you are 30 years old and in perfect health, getting an electrocardiogram to screen for heart disease is a bad idea. So is a mammogram if you're 30 years old and you have nothing wrong with your breasts. And a screening test for HIV infection is worthless if you're in a mutually monogamous relationship, you don't use I.V. drugs and you've never had a blood transfusion.

Deciding which screening tests to have would be much easier if there were a single set of guidelines that all doctors followed. Unfortunately, no such overall set exists (and if it did, many doctors still wouldn't follow it). In fact, different sets of guidelines have sprung up for some individual tests, so doctors will differ in their recommendations about which screening tests you should have, depending on which guidelines they choose to follow.

In some cases, you may be helped in making your decisions about screening tests by the recommendations of reputable organizations like the American Cancer Society, the American College of Obstetricians and Gynecologists or the National Cancer Institute. For example, these organizations have now agreed on uniform guidelines for Pap test screening and mammography. If you are in doubt about a screening procedure your doctor is recommending, consider contacting a national health organization that deals with that particular issue. For example: To decide if your young child should be screened for high blood cholesterol, call or write the American Academy of Pediatrics. (To locate the phone numbers or addresses of an organization, call the reference librarian at your local library or call 1-800-555-1212 to see if the organization has a toll-free number.)

Another source for information on screening guidelines is a book called *Guide To Clinical Preventive Services*, which was written by the U.S. Preventive Services Task Force. (Note: The book is written in rather technical language, since it was intended primarily for use by health care professionals.) In 1989, this Task Force released a report evaluating the cost-effectiveness of a variety of screening tests and other health-related preventive services. In developing this report, the

You can use the Task Force recommendations as a starting point for discussing screening tests and preventive services with your physician.

Task Force reviewed scientific literature and research to determine what the real costs and benefits were for each test and service. After weighing these costs and benefits, the Task Force made recommendations about which tests and preventive services are justified on a routine basis, and which are not.

The Task Force guidelines cover a wide variety of currently recommended tests and services, ranging from screening procedures for heart disease and HIV infection to immunizations and counseling. However, the Task Force recommendations do not necessarily coincide with the guidelines that other groups (such as the American Cancer Society) are making, and which many physicians are following. For example, if a screening test exists for a particular disease, but there are no medical therapies available to cure or treat that disease, the Task Force usually recommended against screening. Following, you will find a summary of the recommendations made by the Task Force. Where these recommendations conflict significantly with the recommendations of other major medical organizations, we have tried to identify the difference.

You can use the Task Force recommendations as a starting point for discussing screening tests and preventive services with your physician. If your doctor recommends a screening test that the Task Force has concluded is unnecessary or not cost-effective, you should ask your doctor to explain why the test may be appropriate in your particular case. Keep in mind that the Task Force recommendations apply to the population at large. Based on your personal medical history and/or physical examination, your doctor may be aware of certain circumstances that justify the use of a particular test or service in your individual case.

SCREENING FOR HEART DISEASE

Blood Pressure Blood pressure should be measured regularly in everyone aged three and above. The pressure should be measured once every two years if the last pressure readings were below 140 systolic and 85 diastolic. If the last diastolic blood pressure was between 85 and 89, the pressure should be measured again within a year. Higher readings require more frequent blood pressure measurements. Hypertension (high blood pressure) should not be diagnosed on the basis of one blood pressure measurement. Elevated pressure readings should be confirmed by multiple measurements at each of three separate visits.

Cholesterol Screening The National Cholesterol Education Program panel recommends that all adults twenty years of age and older have their total blood cholesterol level measured at least once every five years. An HDL cholesterol test should also be conducted at the same time, as long as an accurate measurement can be ensured. For individuals with previously diagnosed coronary heart disease, it is recommended that screenings include measurements of LDL and triglyceride levels as well as the total and HDL levels. For cholesterol levels considered borderline high (200 to 239), individuals are advised to seek more frequent testing of cholesterol levels. If your cholesterol is 240 or greater, a lipoprotein analysis should be ordered, and a cholesterol-lowering program started immediately. Further testing and therapy should be based upon your response to the diet.

Depending on the outcome of these tests—and whether you already have evidence of coronary heart disease and/or any of its risk factors (see box on page 211)—your doctor may provide additional evaluation, guidance and treatment.

Electrocardiograms (also known as EKGs or ECGs) This test measures the electrical activity of your heart, which can tell your doctor if your heart rhythm is normal and may reveal if your heart muscle has been damaged previously by a heart attack. Routine electrocardiograms are not recommended for people under the age of 40 unless they have symptoms that suggest heart disease. Screening electrocardiograms may be advisable in males over age 40 who are free of symptoms if they have any of the following conditions:

- Two or more risk factors for coronary heart disease (see box on following page);

- It would endanger public safety if they had a sudden heart attack (for example, pilots);

- They have been sedentary and are planning to begin a vigorous exercise program.

Routine screening electrocardiograms are not recommended for children, adolescents or young adults who want to enter athletic programs unless they have some evidence suggestive of heart disease.

SCREENING FOR CEREBROVASCULAR DISEASE
(DISEASE OF THE ARTERIES THAT SUPPLY BLOOD TO THE BRAIN)

Your physician should listen with a stethoscope for abnormal sounds over the arteries in the neck under the following conditions:

- In patients with risk factors for cardiovascular disease or cerebrovascular disease, including increased age, elevated blood pressure, high blood cholesterol, atrial fibrillation (an abnormal heart rhythm), a history of smoking and diabetes;

- In all patients who have symptoms suggestive of a nervous system disorder, such as dizziness, fainting spells, seizures or paralysis;

- In anyone who has previously been diagnosed with cerebrovascular disease.

SCREENING FOR PERIPHERAL ARTERY DISEASE
(DISEASE OF THE ARTERIES THAT SUPPLY BLOOD TO THE ARMS & LEGS)

In people with peripheral artery disease, the blood vessels in the arms and legs become narrowed, choking off the flow of blood and oxygen. This condition becomes increasingly common with age, and leads to pain in the legs during walking, ulcers on the skin, and—in severe cases—to gangrene and even loss of the leg.

The risk of peripheral artery disease is greatly increased among smokers and people with diabetes or high blood pressure.

The simplest screening test for peripheral artery disease is to feel the pulses in both wrists and in both feet, and some doctors do this routinely in patients who are at high risk for this problem. But this is not nearly as accurate as measuring the blood pressure in both arms and legs using an ultrasound device. Some "clinics" have been promoting the ultrasound test directly to the public, and some physicians are doing it on most of their older patients. However, because of the expense related to this test, it is not recommended for routine screening, and should be used only in people who have symptoms suggesting peripheral artery disease or abnormalities of their pulses or blood pressure.

SCREENING FOR DIABETES

Diabetes is a condition that causes the blood glucose (sugar) level to rise. If untreated, the abnormally high glucose levels increase the risk of cardiovascular disease, stroke, kidney disease, blindness and many other problems. However, long before these complications occur, the abnormal sugar levels will cause symptoms that should alert physicians to measure blood glucose levels. Therefore, routine screening for diabetes in men and nonpregnant women is not recommended except in selected high-risk groups, including:

- Obese individuals (20 percent or more over ideal weight);
- People with a family history of diabetes;
- Women with a history of diabetes during pregnancy (gestational diabetes).

This screening should take place at the time of a regularly scheduled physical examination. All pregnant women should take a blood test (commonly called the glucose tolerance test) between the 24th and 28th weeks of pregnancy to check for gestational diabetes.

Risk Factors for Coronary Heart Disease

- High Blood Pressure
- Current Cigarette Smoking
- Family History of Coronary Artery Disease (heart attack or sudden death before age 55 in a male parent or sibling, or before age 65 in a female parent or sibling)
- Male Sex (over age 45)
- Female Sex (over age 55, or with premature menopause without estrogen replacement therapy)
- Low HDL Cholesterol (HDL less than 35, confirmed by repeat measurement)
- Non-Insulin-Dependent Diabetes

SCREENING FOR THYROID DISEASE
(OTHER THAN CANCER)

The thyroid gland plays an essential role in regulating metabolism in the body (the rate at which your body creates and uses energy). Thyroid hormones also influence many other processes and organs throughout the body. When the thyroid gland is producing excessive amounts of hormone (hyperthyroidism), many symptoms and physical changes develop, including restlessness, irritability, insomnia, heat intolerance, shortness of breath, diarrhea, weakness, shakiness, rapid heart rate, weight loss and bulging of the eyes. When the gland produces too little hormone (hypothyroidism), the symptoms and physical changes can include confusion, memory loss, weight gain, constipation, hair loss, shortness of breath, numbness, lethargy and inability to tolerate cold temperatures. All of the symptoms listed above can be caused by conditions other than thyroid disease, which explains why the diagnosis is often missed or delayed.

The diagnosis of thyroid disorders is usually made by means of blood tests that measure thyroid hormones and other substances that are affected by thyroid hormones. These tests are very useful in people who have the symptoms noted above, because they help to distinguish those who have thyroid disorders from those who have other problems (for example, weight gain and constipation can be caused by a high-calorie, low-fiber diet, as well as hypothyroidism; and rapid heart rate, insomnia and restlessness can be caused by anxiety, as well as hyperthyroidism). However, the tests are rarely helpful when used to screen people who are in good general health (for example, people who are overweight but otherwise healthy). The only exception to this rule is in newborns, who can develop irreversible mental retardation if hypothyroidism is not detected immediately. Screening for congenital hypothyroidism is recommended for all newborns during the first week of life. Routine screening for thyroid disorders is otherwise not warranted in children or adults, as it has not been proven that adults who are treated before symptoms occur have a better outcome than those whose conditions are detected by screening tests before symptoms occur.

SCREENING FOR LOW BACK PROBLEMS

Some practitioners (most notably, chiropractors) order spinal x-rays routinely to screen people for low back problems. However, these studies are generally not useful, except in people who have suffered specific

> *Because of the radiation exposure associated with spinal x-rays, they should never be used as screening tests in people who are healthy.*

injuries or in whom physical exam suggests that a structural abnormality exists. Because of the radiation exposure associated with spinal x-rays, they should never be used as screening tests in people who are healthy.

SCREENING FOR ANEMIA

Anemia is a disorder related to red blood cells, which are responsible for carrying oxygen throughout the body. In people with anemia, the oxygen-carrying capacity of the blood is decreased because there are too few red blood cells or because their ability to carry oxygen is impaired. There are several different causes of anemia, including hemorrhage (bleeding), iron deficiency and heredity.

Anemia is diagnosed by measuring the number of red cells that are present in a blood specimen or by measuring the amount of hemoglobin present in the red cells. In the past, many physicians performed these blood tests routinely as part of an overall examination. However, studies show that this type of screening is rarely helpful when performed in healthy people. Therefore, these tests should be done only when there are symptoms or physical signs that suggest the possibility that anemia is present (pale skin, rapid pulse, lethargy, shortness of breath), or when there is reason to believe that a person has lost substantial amounts of blood.

The only exceptions to this rule are pregnant women and infants. Hemoglobin analysis (a measure of the major protein in the red blood cell) should be obtained on all pregnant women at their first prenatal visit. Further prenatal testing is not necessary in uncomplicated pregnancies. All infants should be screened once for anemia.

SCREENING FOR BACTERIA, BLOOD AND
PROTEIN IN THE URINE

Testing the Urine for Bacteria In most cases of urinary tract infection, there will be symptoms (fever, frequent urination, pain or burning on urination). However, it is possible for a urinary infection to occur without symptoms, especially in young children, pregnant women, diabetics and the elderly. Therefore, most experts recommend screening for bacteria in the urine in these groups.

The most accurate procedure for detecting bacteria in the urine is a culture test, but this test is time-consuming and expensive. Therefore, most clinicians use a "dipstick" test (a chemically treated paper strip is dipped into the urine specimen; if bacteria are present, the paper strip should change color). If this screening test is positive, a urine culture must be performed to identify exactly which type of bacteria are present (this is done by keeping a specimen of urine warm in an incubator for a day or two to promote growth of any bacteria that are present).

All pregnant women and preschool children should be screened at least once for bacteria in the urine (more often if a physician believes there are other reasons to suspect that bacteria may be present). Diabetics should be screened periodically, with the frequency to be determined by the physician. Since elderly people are also at high risk for urinary infection, periodic screening in this group may be a good idea.

Testing the Urine for Blood and Protein Blood in the urine is often the first sign of cancer in the urinary tract or of serious kidney disease. Blood in the urine may be present in such small amounts that it cannot be seen with the naked eye. In this situation, it can usually be detected by microscopic examination of the urine or by use of a chemically treated strip that is dipped into the urine. Screening the urine for blood and protein is recommended for people over age 60. Your physician will decide how often you should be tested based on your individual medical history.

SCREENING FOR OSTEOPOROSIS

Bone Density Measurements Osteoporosis is a condition in which the bones lose excessive amounts of calcium and thus become more brittle and susceptible to fracture. Among the contributing factors to osteoporosis are calcium deficiency, hereditary susceptibility, lack of estrogen, smoking and sedentary lifestyle. The problem is much more common in women after menopause, because estrogen levels decline (this hormone prevents the loss of calcium from bone).

It is possible to screen for osteoporosis using x-rays of the bone to determine if calcium is being lost. However, routine testing in healthy women is not recommended. It may be justified around the time of menopause in women who are at high risk for osteoporosis to help determine if hormone replacement therapy is appropriate. The following are considered risk factors for osteoporosis:

- Caucasian, Asian, or Indian;
- Small size (less than 5'2" tall, weighing less than 105 pounds) or fair skin;
- A family history of osteoporosis;
- Smoker or long history of prior smoking;
- Sedentary lifestyle;
- Early removal of the ovaries (before menopause).

SCREENING FOR BREAST CANCER

Breast Examination Routine annual breast examination by a health professional is recommended for all women age 40 and above. Women at high risk for breast cancer because of their family history (breast cancer diagnosed before the age of 50 in a mother or sister) should have annual examinations after the age of 35.

Mammography Mammography uses x-rays to identify early signs of breast cancer—before a lump can be felt. Mammography should only be done by experienced radiologists in facilities that have been certified by the American College of Radiology. This is the best way to ensure that you are getting the lowest possible radiation dose, and that the mammograms will be interpreted by a qualified physician.

Mammography is recommended every one to two years for all women beginning at age 50 and concluding at approximately age 75. If

Routine annual breast examination by a health professional is recommended for all women age 40 and above.

abnormalities are found, more frequent testing may be advisable. In women at high risk for breast cancer because of their family history (see above), annual mammography may be a good idea from the age of 40 on. Note: Mammography may be indicated at any age if a woman has breast-related symptoms or abnormalities in the breast on physical examination. The Task Force guidelines differ from those of the American Cancer Society, which recommends a screening mammogram by age 40, a mammogram every one to two years between the age of 40 and 49, and an annual mammogram from age 50 on.

SCREENING FOR CERVICAL CANCER

Pap Exams The Pap smear is obtained by gently scraping cells away from the surface of the cervix. These cells are placed on a glass slide and then examined under a microscope for signs of cancer or precancerous changes. If precancerous changes are detected and the cervix is treated, it is possible to prevent the later development of cancer.

Regular Pap exams are recommended for all women who are (or who have been) sexually active. Testing should begin at the age a woman first engages in sexual intercourse or at age 18, whichever comes first. Pap tests should be performed yearly for three years. If three consecutive annual tests are normal, a three-year interval between Pap exams may be appropriate. A physician may recommend more frequent Pap tests if a woman has any of the following risk factors for cervical cancer:

- Early onset of sexual intercourse;
- A history of multiple sexual partners;
- Low socioeconomic status.

Pap tests may be discontinued at age 65, but only if previous tests have been consistently normal.

SCREENING FOR PROSTATE CANCER

Prostate cancer is the most common cancer in men. The risk of prostate cancer increases with age, beginning around the age of 50 (although, rarely, it does occur earlier). In its earliest stages, while the cancer is still confined to the prostate gland, it rarely produces symptoms. The primary screening tests for diagnosing prostate cancer are digital rectal exam and the PSA (prostate-specific antigen) blood test. During the digital rectal exam, the physician feels the prostate through the rectum for signs of enlargement, lumps, or abnormal hardness. The PSA test looks for increased amounts of a protein that is often manufactured when prostate cancer is present.

Digital Rectal Exam The American Cancer Society recommends that a digital rectal examination be performed annually in all men beginning at age 40.

Prostate Specific Antigen (PSA) The American Cancer Society recommends that men age 50 and older have a yearly blood test to check levels of prostate specific antigen (PSA). The Task Force does not recommend PSA screening, except in men who have signs or symptoms of a prostate abnormality. Their recommendation is based in part on the fact that the PSA is not very accurate, and many men without prostate cancer will have elevated PSA levels, leading to unnecessary concern and, in some cases, unnecessary biopsies of their prostate gland. There is also reason to believe that early detection of this particular kind of cancer does not improve the outcome.

SCREENING FOR TESTICULAR CANCER

Testicular cancer most commonly occurs between the ages of 20 and 35. However, men of any age should seek prompt medical attention if they develop any worrisome symptoms such as testicular pain, swelling or heaviness.

Periodic testicular examinations by a health professional are recommended for men at increased risk of developing testicular cancer. This includes men with a history of any of the following:

> *The American Cancer Society recommends that a digital rectal examination be performed annually in all men beginning at age 40.*

- A testicle that did not descend fully into the scrotum during gestation;

- A testicle that has atrophied (become smaller);

- An operation to attach the testicle to the scrotum (orchiopexy).

How often examinations should be performed needs to be determined on an individual basis in consultation with your physician.

SCREENING FOR COLORECTAL CANCER

Colon cancer is the second-most common cancer in the United States. The long-term survival rate is much better in those who are diagnosed early than for those in whom the cancer is found in later stages.

The primary screening tests for colon cancer include digital rectal examination, fecal occult blood testing and sigmoidoscopy. Rectal examination may detect tumors at the end of the colon, but it cannot identify the presence of any tumors beyond the reach of the examining finger. To examine beyond that point, your doctor must use an instrument (sigmoidoscope or colonoscope) that permits visual examination of the interior surface of the colon. This test is uncomfortable, time-consuming, and expensive. Fecal occult blood testing is based on the fact that colon cancers may cause small amounts of bleeding to occur, even very early in the development of the tumors. Although there may be too little blood present in the stool to visualize with the naked eye, it is possible to detect very tiny amounts with a simple chemical test that your doctor can perform in the office on a stool specimen.

Digital Rectal Examination This procedure should be a part of every complete physical examination your physician performs. The American Cancer Society recommends that it be performed annually starting at age 40. The Task Force recommends this after the age of 50 in people at high risk for colon cancer (see next page).

Occult (Hidden) Blood Testing Testing the stool for hidden blood is controversial, since it has been difficult to prove that this procedure increases the cure rate for colorectal cancer. However, a recent study has demonstrated that the death rate from colon cancer can be cut by 33 percent if the screening test for hidden blood is performed every year (in people who were tested every two years, there was no reduction in overall mortality). The American Cancer Society recommends stool occult blood testing annually for everyone, beginning at age 50. The Task Force recommendation differs, suggesting that routine testing be performed after age 50 only in the following groups of high-risk individuals:

- Those who have an increased risk of developing colon cancer because they have a parent or sibling who had colon cancer;

- Women who have had cancer of the endometrium (the lining of the uterus), breast or ovary;

- People who have previously been diagnosed as having inflammatory bowel disease (ileitis or colitis), adenomatous polyps of the colon or colorectal cancer.

Sigmoidoscopy Periodic sigmoidoscopy (examination of the interior of the colon through a special viewing instrument) is recommended by the American Cancer Society for all people every three to five years, starting at age 50. The Task Force recommends sigmoidoscopy only in persons with a family history of colorectal cancer or colon polyps.

SCREENING FOR LUNG CANCER

Cancer of the lung is the leading cause of cancer deaths in the United States. In the past, screening for lung cancer has been done by examining chest x-rays and sputum cytology specimens (like the Pap smear, this involves microscopically examining cells from the surface of the breathing tubes that are coughed up with sputum). However, there is little evidence that screening for lung cancer this way reduces the mortality from this disease. Therefore, routine screening for lung cancer is not recommended.

SCREENING FOR SKIN CANCER

Skin cancer is the most common cancer in the United States (more than 500,000 new cases are diagnosed every year). Although skin cancers are easily treated and highly curable when diagnosed early, they can be very disfiguring and even life-threatening when allowed to progress (skin cancer accounts for more than 2,000 deaths per year).

The principal screening test for skin cancer is physical examination of the skin. You can perform this test yourself in front of a full-length mirror, looking for the following: any change in the color, size or shape of a mole; sores or lesions that crust, bleed or fail to heal. The American Academy of Dermatology and the American Cancer Society recommend an annual complete skin examination by a physician (complete skin examination should be a part of any complete routine physical examination your doctor performs). The Task Force recommends such examinations only for people who are at high risk of developing skin cancer, including:

- People with a family history of skin cancer;
- Individuals with a previous cancerous skin lesion;
- People with increased occupational or recreational exposure to sunlight (e.g., lifeguard);
- People with precancerous skin lesions (abnormal moles, solar keratoses).

How often these examinations are performed should be tailored to the needs of the individual by the supervising physician.

SCREENING FOR OVARIAN CANCER

Although not one of the most common cancers, ovarian cancer is one of the most lethal in women, accounting for more than 10,000 deaths per year. The primary potential screening tests for ovarian cancer include pelvic examination by a health professional, blood testing for CA 125 (a protein that is increased in some patients with ovarian cancer) and ultrasound examination of the pelvis. None of these procedures is very accurate for making the diagnosis of ovarian cancer.

Pelvic Examination A pelvic exam can reveal when an ovary is enlarged, but other procedures—usually involving surgery—are necessary to determine if the enlargement is due to cancer or the result of a benign process. The American College of Obstetricians and Gynecologists and the American Cancer Society recommend an annual pelvic examination, which includes examination of the ovaries (Note: Pap tests are not necessarily done at every exam). The Task Force does not recommend

> *Colon cancer is the second-most common cancer in the United States. The long-term survival rate is much better in those who are diagnosed early than for those in whom the cancer is found in later stages.*

that ovarian exams be done more frequently than the recommended interval for Pap tests, unless there are other medical reasons for an examination.

CA 125 Blood Test This test is not recommended for routine screening because of its low level of accuracy. The CA 125 level can be abnormally high in people without cancer or in women with benign (noncancerous) problems of their ovaries. Also, it can be normal in women who have ovarian cancer.

Pelvic Ultrasound This test is not recommended for routine screening because it is expensive and has a low level of accuracy. Ultrasound testing produces false positive results in a significant percentage of women with healthy ovaries, leading them to undergo additional testing that is risky, expensive and unnecessary.

SCREENING FOR PANCREATIC CANCER

Routine screening for pancreatic cancer is not recommended, as the potential tests for this purpose (ultrasound, blood test, CT scans) are expensive and lack the accuracy necessary for reliability.

SCREENING FOR ORAL CANCER

Everyone, but particularly those over age 65, should have regular dental examinations (the American Dental Association recommends hav-

> *Everyone, but particularly those over age 65, should have regular dental examinations.*

ing checkups twice a year). A complete oral examination should be performed at each dental visit, looking for any signs of cancer or precancerous lesions. Regular examinations are especially important in people with risk factors predisposing them to oral cancer. This includes people who smoke or chew tobacco or who drink excessive amounts of alcohol, as well as people with suspicious sores in the mouth.

SCREENING FOR TUBERCULOSIS

The skin test for tuberculosis infection, the Mantoux skin test, should be performed on all people at increased risk of developing tuberculosis. This includes:

- Household members of people with tuberculosis;

- People in close contact with individuals with tuberculosis (e.g., medical personnel or nursing home staff members);

- Recent immigrants or refugees from countries where tuberculosis is common (e.g., Asia, Africa, Central and South America, Pacific Islands, the Caribbean);

- Migrant workers;

- Residents of nursing homes, correctional institutions and homeless shelters;

- People with medical conditions that reduce resistance to tuberculosis (HIV infection, immune disorders).

SCREENING FOR RUBELLA (GERMAN MEASLES)

Rubella is a viral infection that generally causes a rash and swollen lymph nodes; this infection can result in serious problems if a woman is infected during pregnancy.

Blood testing for rubella antibodies should be performed in all pregnant and nonpregnant women of childbearing age (except in those already known to be immune because of prior infection or immunization). Nonimmune, nonpregnant women who agree not to become pregnant for three months should be vaccinated. Nonimmune pregnant women should not be vaccinated until immediately after delivery.

Routine screening for rubella is not recommended for men.

SCREENING FOR HEPATITIS B

Hepatitis B is a viral infection affecting the liver that is most commonly transmitted through blood, contaminated needles and intimate contact. Additionally, it can be transmitted to a fetus while in utero or at the time of delivery if the mother is infected.

All pregnant women should be tested for hepatitis B at their first prenatal visit. Testing can be repeated during the third trimester in women who have any of the following risk factors for hepatitis:

- Intravenous drug abuse;
- Heterosexual contact with a person who is infected with hepatitis B;
- Multiple sexual partners.

Routine screening for hepatitis B is not recommended for men and nonpregnant women.

SCREENING FOR HIV INFECTION

It is estimated that 1–1.5 million persons in the United States are infected with the human immunodeficiency virus (HIV, the virus that causes AIDS). A blood screening test for antibodies against HIV will reveal when an infection is present. However, it often takes up to 6–12 weeks after a person is infected before the test will turn positive. Screening for HIV infection is recommended for anyone in the following groups:

- Persons seeking treatment for sexually transmitted diseases;
- Persons who have had multiple sexual partners;
- Intravenous drug users;
- Homosexual and bisexual men;
- Women whose past or present sexual partners were HIV-infected, bisexual or intravenous drug users;

- People with long-term residence or birth in an area with a high prevalence of HIV;

- Individuals who received a blood transfusion between 1978 and 1985.

Testing should also be offered to pregnant women (or women thinking about becoming pregnant) who are at high risk for HIV infection.

SCREENING FOR SYPHILIS

Syphilis is a sexually transmitted disease caused by bacteria. If syphilis is left untreated, it can eventually cause very serious neurologic and cardiovascular complications. Routine blood testing for syphilis is recommended for both men and women with any of the following risk factors:

- People who engage in sex with multiple partners in geographic areas where syphilis is prevalent;

- Sexual partners of people with syphilis;

- Prostitutes.

In addition, all pregnant women should be tested at their first prenatal visit and again at the time of delivery. Women at high risk of acquiring syphilis during their pregnancy (see risk factors noted above) should also be tested at 28 weeks gestation.

SCREENING FOR GONORRHEA

Gonorrhea is a sexually transmitted disease caused by bacteria. The screening test for gonorrhea infection involves taking a specimen from the urethra in men or from the cervix in women for culture in the laboratory (the specimen is kept warm for a day or two and then microscopically examined for evidence of bacterial growth). Routine cultures for gonorrhea should be obtained in the following high-risk groups of men and women:

- People with multiple sexual partners or a sexual partner with multiple sexual partners;

- Individuals who have had sexual contact with people who have gonorrhea;

- People with a history of repeated bouts of gonorrhea;

- Prostitutes.

Pregnant women should have gonorrhea cultures at their first prenatal visit. Testing later in pregnancy is recommended for women at high risk (see risk factors noted above) of contracting gonorrhea during their pregnancy.

SCREENING FOR CHLAMYDIA

Chlamydia is a sexually transmitted disease caused by bacteria. Screening for chlamydia infection can be accomplished by culture or blood testing. Routine testing for chlamydia infections is recommended for the following high-risk groups:

- Sexually active teenagers;

- People with multiple sexual partners;

- People who have a partner who has multiple sexual partners;

- Recent sexual partners of individuals that have chlamydial infections;

- People being treated for other sexually transmitted diseases.

Pregnant women in the high-risk categories listed above should be tested for chlamydia at their first prenatal visit.

SCREENING FOR GENITAL HERPES SIMPLEX

Genital herpes is a sexually transmitted disease caused by a virus. Screening for this disease can be done through viral cultures taken from active sores or the genital area. This test is reliable when lesions are present, but much less so in the absence of active infection. Routine screening for genital herpes is not recommended for men and nonpregnant women. Screening is recommended for pregnant women with active herpes lesions, but is not necessary in the absence of active disease.

SCREENING FOR LEAD TOXICITY

Excessive lead in the body can lead to a variety of serious complications in both children and adults. Children are at special risk because high levels of lead in the blood can cause nervous system damage and lowering of the intelligence quotient (I.Q.). Annual blood testing of lead screening is recommended for all children aged nine months to six years who are at high risk for lead toxicity. Even more frequent screening is recommended in some urban areas such as New York City, where levels of lead in the environment are high. Call your local health department to find the recommended frequency for screening in your area. High risk groups include:

- Children who live in or who frequently visit older housing that is run down or undergoing renovation;

- Children who come in close contact with children with known lead toxicity;

- Children living near lead processing plants or whose parents work in a lead-related occupation;

- Children living near busy highways or hazardous waste sites.

Routine annual screening of older children and adults is not necessary except when lead exposure is suspected, or in urban areas where environmental lead levels are thought to be high.

VISION SCREENING

Vision screening (eye charts) is recommended for all children once before entering school, preferably at the age of three or four. While routine vision testing is not recommended in schoolchildren without signs of visual problems or bad eyesight, doctors should be alert for signs of ocular misalignment (where one eye turns in or out, or fails to follow the other eye's movements). Vision screening of adolescents and adults is not recommended by the Task Force. However, the American Academy of Ophthalmology recommends eye exams at least every 2 to 4 years after the age of 40.

SCREENING FOR GLAUCOMA

Glaucoma is a condition that causes the pressure within the eyeball to rise to abnormally high levels. It is the second leading cause of new cases of blindness in the United States. The screening test for glaucoma is called tonometry, which uses a device placed on the cornea or a puff of air blown against the cornea to measure the pressure inside the eye. Routine testing for glaucoma by primary care physicians is not advocated.

For those at high risk of developing glaucoma, testing should be done periodically by an eye specialist. The American Academy of Ophthalmology recommends testing every three to five years before the age of 40 if you have any of the following risk factors for glaucoma:

- A family history of the disease;
- History of an eye injury;
- African-American descent.

Starting at age 40, the Academy recommends that everyoine (whether they're considered at risk or not) undergo a complete eye examination (including testing for glaucoma) once every two to four years. After the age of 65, these examinations should be performed more frequently, at least once every one to two years.

SCREENING FOR HEARING IMPAIRMENT

Screening should be performed on all newborns at high risk for hearing impairment. This is done by observing how the child reacts to noise and, if necessary, by actually measuring the infant's brain wave reactions to noise. Risk factors include:

- A family history of childhood hearing impairment; infection with herpes, syphilis, rubella, cytomegalovirus or toxoplasmosis in utero or shortly after birth;
- Congenital malformations of the head or neck;
- Low birthweight (less than 1,500 grams or 3.3 pounds);
- Bacterial meningitis;
- High levels of bilirubin in the blood at birth (jaundice);
- Inadequate oxygenation around the time of birth.

High-risk infants who are not tested at birth should be tested before the age of three.

Screening is recommended for adolescents and adults only if they are routinely exposed to loud noise. Elderly patients should have their hearing routinely evaluated and should be counseled about the availability and use of hearing aids.

SCREENING FOR INTRAUTERINE GROWTH RETARDATION (FAILURE OF A FETUS TO GROW PROPERLY)

Pregnant women at increased risk for intrauterine growth retardation (IUGR—abnormally slow growth and small size of the baby) should have ultrasound examinations of their fetus in the second trimester to determine its correct age and again in the third trimester to measure the size of important fetal structures. Women at risk for IUGR include:

- Women with high blood pressure;
- Women with kidney disease;
- Women who are short;
- Women who smoke, drink alcohol or abuse other drugs;
- Women with a history of a previous pregnancy with growth retardation or fetal death.
- Women who have a low prepregnancy weight or who fail to gain weight during pregnancy.

Routine ultrasound testing is otherwise not recommended in normal pregnancies.

SCREENING FOR CONGENITAL BIRTH DEFECTS

Several tests can be used during pregnancy to determine if abnormalities are present in the fetus. These include examination of the fetal genetic material (chromosome analysis); chemical tests for evidence of protein abnormalities associated with certain problems and ultrasound examination to detect overt physical deformities.

Amniocentesis Amniocentesis for chromosomal analysis should be offered to pregnant women aged 35 and older. In younger women, amniocentesis is unnecessary unless there are special indications.

Alpha-fetoprotein Alpha-fetoprotein levels should be measured in pregnant women between weeks 16 and 18 of pregnancy. High levels of this protein in the blood of a pregnant woman suggest the possibility of fetal abnormalities of the spinal cord or brain.

Ultrasound Ultrasound examinations are not recommended as a routine screening test for birth defects.

RESOURCES

Information is empowering. The more you know about the health care marketplace and about any illnesses you or your family members may have, the better equipped you'll be to get the best possible treatment without overspending.

So where should you look for information about the health problems that afflict your family? Let's take a closer look at some of the best resources.

Libraries

The ideal place to start is at the public library nearest you. Besides having books available on a wide variety of health topics—from arthritis to allergies—the library can often obtain books for you that aren't already on its own shelves through an interlibrary loan system. It might take a few days or even several weeks to track down the book you want, but if you're patient, you can get it on loan free of charge.

Also, don't overlook the medical libraries at hospitals and at the school of public health at universities in your area. Although these libraries and their staff exist primarily to serve physicians and students, most make their materials available to the public, as well, usually without charge. In particular, these libraries tend to have good collections of medical journals. If you need more technical information than you're finding at a public library, visit a local hospital and ask the librarian there for help in locating relevant journal articles.

Incidentally, audio and videotapes on health topics are becoming nearly as popular as books. Not only do some libraries stock these

The more you know about the health care marketplace and about any illnesses you or your family members may have, the better equipped you'll be to get the best possible treatment without overspending.

tapes, but so do many video stores. At the major video chains, you can often rent these items for a couple of dollars a night—or, in some cases, even borrow them at no cost.

Voluntary Organizations

Name a disease, and there's probably a voluntary organization to support those affected by it. Most people are familiar with organizations such as the American Cancer Society, the American Heart Association and the American Diabetes Association. But there are hundreds of others, from the American Chronic Pain Association to the National Association for Sickle Cell Disease to the National Osteoporosis Foundation.

Most of these organizations were founded by people suffering from that particular disorder. Their goals are usually to support research in the field and to educate the public about that disorder or disease. While many organizations have salaried staff members, most of the manpower is supplied by volunteers with a personal connection to—and a commitment to eradicating—the disorder.

Our own experience has led us to a simple conclusion: If you make use of the services of these organizations, they can dramatically change your life. They gather and disseminate reliable, thorough and up-to-date information about diseases and their treatments. They can refer you to research sites, experts in the field and relevant scientific literature. And, they can put you on the road to personally conquering an illness—or at least learning to live more successfully with it.

SUPPORT GROUPS

Voluntary organizations, especially their local chapters, can provide another important service: They can put you in touch with support groups in your community. We can't overemphasize the value of such support. No one understands an illness or a problem better than someone who has it. As sympathetic and compassionate as a caring doctor or family members may be, the person who is ill will frequently tell them (or would like to tell them), "You can't possibly know what it's really like to have this problem." And it's the truth.

> *Recent studies have shown that the support of others is not only emotionally nourishing, but it may actually improve a patient's physical condition.*

But support groups are different. The people who participate in them have a shared condition, and together they can discuss mutual concerns and anxieties, as well as compare notes on their encounters with both traditional and alternative therapies. In the process, participants can end their sense of isolation or alienation, draw strength from one another, and learn to better cope with their life situation.

Just how valuable are these support groups? Recent studies have shown that the support of others is not only emotionally nourishing, but it may actually improve a patient's physical condition. Consider the findings of a study at Stanford University. Psychiatrist David Spiegel and his associates found that when advanced breast cancer patients participated in support groups along with hypnosis and relaxation therapy, they lived an average of 18 months longer than did women who did not take part in group therapy.

If you have a chronic illness, we urge you to find and participate in a support group in your area. If a voluntary organization can't put you in touch with other patients with the same disease or condition, contact the American Self-Help Clearinghouse (St. Clares-Riverside Medical Center, 25 Pocono Road, Denville, NJ 07834; 201-625-7101) for assistance.

Most support groups convene weekly or biweekly in private homes or in hospital meeting rooms. There's often no fee to participate, although there might be a small charge to help pay for rental of the meeting room. It's money well spent, for you may soon find that a support group can not only improve the quality of your life, but perhaps help in the healing process, too.

A List of Resources

There are 5,000 to 10,000 diseases that go by a total of about 20,000 names. We simply don't have the space in this book to provide names, addresses and phone numbers for all the organizations concerned with these conditions. But the following list represents the most common problems and disorders. We have limited our listings to those that can directly impact the cost of medical care by providing free or low-cost information, referrals and other services. At the time of publication, we made special efforts to ensure the accuracy of these listings, but bear in mind that addresses and phone numbers are subject to change.

If you don't find a listing for a particular condition, especially if it's an uncommon disorder, contact the National Organization for Rare Disorders (P.O. Box 8923, New Fairfield, CT 06812; 800-447-6673). Its staff should be able to help you locate the most relevant organization.

For more detailed information regarding consumer health insurance problems in your area, there is a list of State Insurance Offices, with addresses and phone numbers, appearing at the end of this section.

ORGANIZATIONS

ADRENAL DISEASES

> National Adrenal Diseases Foundation
> 505 Northern Boulevard
> Great Neck, NY 11021
> (516) 487-4992

AGING

> The Administration On Aging,
> Department of Health and Human Services,
> operates a referral service to help identify
> community services available to the elderly.
> They can be contacted at (800) 677-1116.

> American Association Of Retired Persons
> 601 E Street, N.W.
> Washington, D.C. 20049
> (800) 453-5800

Children Of Aging Parents
1609 Woodbourne Road, Suite 302A
Levittown, PA 19057
(215) 945-6900

Eldercare Locator
(800) 677-1116

National Council On The Aging
409 Third Street, S.W.
2nd Floor
Washington, D.C. 20024
(800) 292-3513
(202) 479-1200

National Institute On Aging Information Center
P.O. Box 8057
Gaithersburg, MD 20898-8057
(800) 222-2225
(301) 587-2528

AIDS

AIDS Hotline For Teens
(800) 234-8336

American Social Health Association
P.O. Box 13827
Research Triangle Park, NC 27709
(919) 361-8400

Information On Experimental Drugs
(800) 822-7422

National AIDS Hotline
(800) 342-2437
(800) 344-7432 (Spanish)

National AIDS Information Clearinghouse
P.O. Box 6003
Rockville, MD 20849-6003
(800) 458-5231

Pediatric AIDS Foundation
1311 Colorado Avenue
Santa Monica, CA 90404
(310) 395-9051

ALLERGIES

Allergy and Asthma Network/Mothers of Asthmatics, Inc.
3554 Chain Bridge Road, Suite 200
Fairfax, VA 22030
(800) 878-4403
(703) 385-4403

American Academy Of Allergy And Immunology
611 East Wells Street
Milwaukee, WI 53202
(800) 822-2762
(414) 272-6071

American Allergy Association
P.O. Box 7273
Menlo Park, CA 94026
(415) 322-1663

Asthma And Allergy Foundation Of America
1125 Fifteenth Street, N.W., Suite 502
Washington, D.C. 20005
(800) 727-8462
(202) 466-7643

National Institute Of Allergy And Infectious Diseases
Office of Communications
Building 31, Room 7A50
9000 Rockville Pike
Bethesda, MD 20892
(301) 496-5717

ALZHEIMER'S DISEASE

Alzheimer's Association
919 North Michigan Avenue, Suite 1000
Chicago, IL 60611-1676
(800) 272-3900

Alzheimer's Disease Education
And Referral Center
P.O. Box 825
Silver Spring, MD 20907-8250
(800) 438-4380

American Health Assistance Foundation
15825 Shady Grove Road, Suite 140
Rockville, MD 20850
(800) 437-2423

AMYOTROPHIC LATERAL SCLEROSIS

ALS Association
21021 Ventura Boulevard
Woodland Hills, CA 9136
(800) 782-4747
(818) 340-7500

ARTHRITIS

Arthritis Foundation
P.O. Box 19000
Atlanta, GA 30326
(800) 283-7800
(404) 872-7100

National Institute Of Arthritis And
Musculoskeletal And Skin Diseases
Building 31, Room 4C05
9000 Rockville Pike
Bethesda, MD 20892
(301) 496-8188

ASTHMA

Allergy And Asthma Network/
Mothers of Asthmatics, Inc.
3554 Chain Bridge Road, Suite 200
Fairfax, VA 22030
(800) 878-4403
(703) 385-4403

Asthma And Allergy Foundation Of America
1125 Fifteenth Street, N.W.
Suite 502
Washington, D.C. 20005
(800) 727-8462
(202) 466-7643

Asthma Information Center Hotline
(800) 727-5400

AUTISM

Autism Society Of America
7910 Woodmont Avenu
 Suite 650
Bethesda, MD 20814
(301) 565-0433

National Autism Hotline
P.O. Box 507
Huntington, WV 25710-0507
(304) 525-8014

BIRTH DEFECTS

Association Of Birth Defect Children, Inc.
5400 Diplomat Circle, Suite 270
Orlando, FL 32810
(407) 629-1466

March Of Dimes Birth Defects Foundation
1275 Mamaroneck Avenue
White Plains, NY 10605
(914) 428-7100

BURNS

The Phoenix Society For Burn Survivors
11 Rust Hill Road
Levittown, PA 19056
(800) 888-2876
(215) 946-2876

CANCER

American Cancer Society, National Office
1599 Clifton Road, N.E.
Atlanta, GA 30329
(800) 227-2345
(404) 320-3333

National Cancer Care Foundation
1180 Avenue of the Americas
New York, NY 10036
(212) 221-3300

National Cancer Institute
Cancer Information Service
Office of Cancer Communications
Building 31, Room 10A24
9000 Rockville Pike
Bethesda, MD 20892
(800) 422-6237 (Bilingual)
(800) 524-1234 (Hawaii only)
(800) 638-6070 (Alaska only)

Rose Kushner Breast Cancer Advisory Center
P.O. Box 224
Kensington, MD 20895
(301) 949-2531

Y-ME National Organization For Breast
Cancer Information And Support
18220 Harwood Avenue
Homewood, IL 60430
(800) 221-2141

CEREBRAL PALSY

United Cerebral Palsy Associations, Inc.
1522 K Street, N.W., Suite 1112
Washington, D.C. 20005-1202
(800) 872-5827
(202) 842-1266

CHILD ABUSE

Child Help USA Hotline
(800) 422-4453

Clearinghouse For Child Abuse And Neglect Information
P.O. Box 1182
Washington, D.C. 20013
(800) 394-3366

CHRONIC FATIGUE SYNDROME

The CFIDS Association Of America, Inc.
P.O. Box 220398
Charlotte, NC 28222-0398
(800) 442-3437
(900) 896-2343

CLEFT PALATE

American Cleft Palate Foundation
1218 Grandview Avenue
Pittsburgh, PA 15211
(800) 242-5338
(412) 481-1376

COOLEY'S ANEMIA

Cooley's Anemia Foundation
105 East 22nd Street
New York, NY 10010
(800) 221-3571
(212) 598-0911

CYSTIC FIBROSIS

Cystic Fibrosis Foundation
6931 Arlington Road
Bethesda, MD 20814
(800) 344-4823
(301) 951-4422
Mail Order Pharmacy (800) 541-4959
Home Health Care (800) 342-6967

DENTAL HEALTH

American Dental Association
211 East Chicago Avenue
Chicago, IL 60611-2678
(312) 440-2500

National Institute Of Dental Research
Building 31, Room 2C35
9000 Rockville Pike
Bethesda, MD 20892
(301) 496-4261

DIABETES

American Diabetes Association
National Center
1600 Duke Street
Alexandria, VA 22314
(800) 232-3472
(703) 549-1500

Juvenile Diabetes Foundation
432 Park Avenue, S., 16th Floor
New York, NY 10016
(800) 223-1138
(212) 889-7575

DISABILITIES

Information Center For Individuals With Disabilities
Fort Point Place
27-43 Wormwood Street
Boston, MA 02210
(800) 462-5015
(617) 727-5540

National Center For Children And Youth With Disabilities
P.O. Box 1492
Washington, D.C. 20013-1492
(703) 893-6061

National Easter Seal Society
230 W. Monroe Street, Suite 1800
Chicago, IL 60606
(312) 726-6200
(312) 726-4258 (TDD)

National Information Clearinghouse For Infants With
Disabilities And Life-threatening Conditions
NISCDD/USC
Benson Boulevard
First Floor
Columbia, SC 29208
(800) 922-9234

National Organization On Disability
910 16th Street, N.W.
Suite 600
Washington, D.C. 20005
(800) 248-2253

National Rehabilitation Information Center
8455 Colesville Road
Suite 935
Silver Spring, MD 20910-3319
(800) 346-2742

DOWN'S SYNDROME

National Down's Syndrome Congress
1800 Dempster Street
Park Ridge, IL 60068-1146
(800) 232-6372
(708) 823-7550

National Down's Syndrome Society
666 Broadway
Room 810
New York, NY 10012
(800) 221-4602
(212) 460-9330

DRUG AND ALCOHOL ABUSE

Al-Anon/Alateen Family Group Headquarters, Inc.
P.O. Box 862
Midtown Station
New York, NY 10018-0862
(800) 344-2666
(212) 302-7240

Alcoholics Anonymous
Grand Central Station
475 Riverside Drive
New York, NY 10115
(212) 870-3400

American Council For Drug Education
204 Monroe Street, Suite 110
Rockville, MD 20850
(800) 488-3784
(301) 294-0600

American Council On Alcoholism
5024 Campbell Boulevard,
Suite H
Baltimore, MD 21236
(800) 527-5344
(410) 931-9393

Drug Abuse Referral Helpline
(800) 622-4357
(800-662-9832) Spanish

National Clearinghouse For Alcohol And Drug Information
P.O. Box 2345
Rockville, MD 20847-2345
(800) 729-6686

National Council On Alcohol And Drugs
(Referrals To Affiliates In Caller's Geographic Area)
(800) 475-4673

National Drug Abuse Information And Treatment Hotline
(800) 662-4357

National Institute On Drug Abuse
Treatment Referral Hotline
(800) 475-4357

National Cocaine Hotline
P.O. Box 100
Summit NJ 07901
(800) 262-2463

DYSLEXIA

Orton Dyslexia Society
Chester Building
Suite 382
8600 LaSalle Road
Baltimore, MD 21204-6020
(800) 222-3123
(410) 296-0232

EATING DISORDERS

American Anorexia/Bulimia Association, Inc.
418 East 76th Street, #3B
New York, NY 10021
(212) 734-1114

Anorexia Nervosa And Related Eating Disorders, Inc.
P.O. Box 5102
Eugene, OR 97405
(503) 344-1144
5238 Duvall Drive
Bethesda, MD 20816
(301) 229-6904

National Anorexic Aid Society
Harding Hospital
445 E. Granville Road
Worthington, OH 43085
(614) 436-1112

National Association Of Anorexia Nervosa
And Associated Disorders
P.O. Box 7
Highland Park, IL 60035
(708) 831-3438

Overeaters Anonymous
P.O. Box 92870
Los Angeles, CA 90009
(310) 618-8835

ENDOMETRIOSIS

Endometriosis Association
8585 N. 76th Place
Milwaukee, WI 53223
(800) 992-3636
(414) 355-2200

EPILEPSY

Epilepsy Foundation Of America
4351 Garden City Drive, Suite 406
Landover, MD 20785
(800) 332-1000
(301) 459-3700

FAMILY PLANNING

Planned Parenthood Federation Of America, Inc.
Educational Resources Clearinghouse
Library and Information Network
810 Seventh Avenue
New York, NY 10019
(800) 230-7526
(212) 541-7800

FANCONI'S ANEMIA

Fanconi's Anemia Research Fund
66 Club Road
Suite 390
Eugene, OR 97401
(503) 687-4658

GASTROINTESTINAL DISEASE

Crohn's And Colitis Foundation Of America, Inc.
444 Park Avenue South, 11th Floor
New York, NY 10016-7374
(800) 343-3637
(212) 685-3440

National Digestive Diseases Information Clearinghouse
Box NDDIC
9000 Rockville Pike
Bethesda, MD 20892
(301) 468-6344

National Foundation For Ileitis And Colitis
444 Park Avenue, 11th Floor
New York, NY 10016
(800) 932-2423
(212) 685-3440

United Ostomy Association
36 Executive Park
Suite 120
Irvine, CA 92714
(800) 826-0826
(714) 660-8624

GENETIC DISORDERS

Alliance Of Genetic Support Groups
35 Wisconsin Circle, Suite 440
Chevy Chase, MD 20815
(800) 336-4363
(301) 652-5553

GUILLAIN-BARRE SYNDROME

Guillain-Barre Syndrome Foundation International
P.O. Box 262
Wynnewood, PA 19096
(215) 667-0131

HEADACHE

National Headache Foundation
5252 North Western Avenue
Chicago, IL 60625
(800) 843-2256
(312) 878-7715

HEAD INJURY

National Head Injury Foundation
1776 Massachusetts Avenue, N.W.
Suite 100
Washington, D.C. 20036
(800) 444-6443
(202) 296-6443

HEALTH INSURANCE

Health Insurance Association Of America
(800) 942-4242
(Note: This helpline is sponsored by the insurance industry.)

HEARING LOSS/DEAFNESS

American Speech-Language-Hearing Association
10801 Rockville Pike
Rockville, MD 20852
(800) 638-8255
(301) 897-5700

Better Hearing Institute
P.O. Box 1840
Washington, D.C. 20013
(800) 327-9355

The Deafness Research Foundation
9 E. 38th Street
New York, NY 10016
(800) 535-3323
(212) 684-6556

Dial-A-Hearing Screening Test
Occupational Hearing Services
300 South Chester Road
Swarthmore, PA 19081
(800) 222-3277

Hear Now
National Hearing Aid Bank
9745 E. Hampden, Suite 300
Denver, CO 80231-4923
(800) 648-4327

National Information Center On Deafness
Gallaudet University
800 Florida Avenue, NE
Washington, D.C. 20002
(202) 651-5051 (Voice)
(202) 651-5052 (TDD)

National Institute On Deafness And Other Communication
Disorders Information Clearinghouse
1010 Wayne Avenue, Suite 300
Silver Spring, MD 20910
(800) 241-1044
(800) 241-1055 (TT)
(301) 565-4020

Self-Help For Hard Of Hearing People, Inc.
7800 Wisconsin Avenue
Bethesda, MD 20814
(301) 657-2248 (Voice)
(301) 657-2249 (TDD)

Tripod Grapevine
2901 North Keystone Street
Burbank, CA 91504
(800) 352-8888 (Voice/TDD)
(800) 287-4763 (Voice/TDD)
(818) 972-2080 (Voice/TDD)

HEART DISEASE

American Heart Association
7272 Greenville Avenue
Dallas, TX 75231-4596
(800) 242-8721
(214) 373-6300

National Heart, Lung, and Blood Institute
Education Programs Information Center
P.O. Box 30105
Bethesda, MD 20824-0105
(301) 251-1122

The Mended Hearts, Inc.
7272 Greenville Avenue
Dallas, TX 75231-4596
(214) 706-1442

HEMOPHILIA

National Hemophilia Foundation
110 Greene Street, Suite 406
New York, NY 10012
(800) 424-2634
(212) 431-8541

HISTIOCYTOSIS

Histiocytosis Association Of America
609 New York Road
Glassboro, NJ 08028
(800) 548-2758
(609) 881-4911

HOME CARE

National Association For Home Care
519 C Street, NE
Washington, D.C. 20002-5809
(202) 547-7424

Visiting Nurse Associations Of America
3801 E. Florida Avenue
Suite 900
Denver, CO 80210
(800) 426-2547

HOSPICE

Children's Hospice International
700 Princess Street
Lower Level
Alexandria, VA 22314-2265
(800) 242-4453

Hospice Association Of America
519 C Street, NE
Washington, D.C. 20002
(202) 546-4759

Hospice Link
Hospice Education Institute
5 Essex Square
Suite 3B
P.O. Box 713
Essex, CT 06426
(800) 331-1620
(203) 767-1620

HOSPITAL CARE

Hill-Burton Free Care Program
Department of Health and
Human Services
(800) 638-0742

Shriner's Hospital Referral Line
P.O. Box 31356
Tampa, FL 33631-3356
(800) 237-5055
(800) 282-9161 (Florida only)

HUNTINGTON'S DISEASE

Huntington's Disease Society of America
140 W. 22nd Street
6th Floor
New York, NY 10011-2420
(800) 345-4372
(212) 242-1968

HYPERTENSION

National High Blood Pressure Education Program
P.O. Box 30105
Bethesda, MD 20824-0105
(301) 251-1222

National Hypertension Association
324 E. 30th Street
New York, NY 10016
(212) 889-3557

HYDROCEPHALUS

Hydrocephalus Association
2040 Polk Street
Room 342
San Francisco, CA 94109
(415) 776-4713

National Hydrocephalus Foundation
400 N. Michigan Avenue
Suite 1102
Chicago, IL 60611-4102
(815) 467-6548

HYSTERECTOMY

Hysterectomy Educational Resources And
Services Foundation
422 Bryn Mawr Avenue
Bala Cynwyd, PA 19004
(215) 667-7757

IMPOTENCE

Impotence Information Center
Minneapolis, MN
(800) 843-4315

Impotence World Services
119 South Ruth Street
Maryville, TN 37801
(615) 983-6092

INCONTINENCE

Help For Incontinent Patients
P.O. Box 8306
Spartanburg, SC 29305
(800) 252-3337

Simon Foundation
P.O. Box 815
Willmette, IL 60091
(800) 237-4666

INFERTILITY

Resolve, Inc.
1310 Broadway
Somerville, MA 02144-1731
(617) 623-0744 (HelpLine)
(617) 623-1156 (Business Office)

The American Fertility Society
1209 Montgomery Highway
Birmingham, AL 35216-2809
(205) 978-5000

INTERSTITIAL CYSTITIS

Interstitial Cystitis Association
P.O. Box 1553, Madison Square Station
New York, NY 10159
(800) 435-7422
(212) 979-6057

KIDNEY DISEASE

American Association Of Kidney Patients
111 S. Parker Street
Suite 405
Tampa, FL 33612
(800) 749-2257
(813) 251-0725

American Kidney Fund
6110 Executive Blvd.
Suite 1010
Rockville, MD 20852
(800) 638-8299
(301) 881-3052

The National Kidney And Urologic
Diseases Information Clearinghouse
P.O. Box NKUDIC
9000 Rockville Pike
Rockville, MD 20892
(301) 468-6345

National Kidney Foundation
30 East 33rd Street, 11th Floor
New York, NY 10016
(800) 622-9010
(212) 889-2210

LEARNING DISABILITIES

Learning Disabilities Association Of America
4156 Library Road
Pittsburgh, PA 15234
(412) 341-1515

National Center For Learning Disabilities
381 Park Avenue South
Suite 1420
New York, NY 10016
(212) 687-7211

LEUKEMIA

The Leukemia Society Of America
600 Third Avenue
New York, NY 10016
(800) 955-4572
(212) 573-8484

LIVER DISEASE

American Liver Foundation
1425 Pompton Avenue
Cedar Grove, NJ 07009
(800) 223-0179
(201) 256-2550

LUNG DISEASE

American Lung Association
1740 Broadway
New York, NY 10019-4374
(212) 315-8700

National Heart, Lung And Blood Institute
Education Programs Information Center
P.O. Box 30105
Bethesda, MD 20824-0105
(301) 951-3260

National Jewish Center For Immunology
And Respiratory Medicine
1400 Jackson Street
Denver, CO 80206
Lungline 800-222-5864
(303) 388-4461

LUPUS

Lupus Support Club
8039 Nova Court
North Charleston, SC 29420
(803) 764-1769

Lupus Foundation Of America, Inc.
4 Research Place
Suite 180
Rockville, MD 20850-3226
(800) 558-0121
(800) 558-0231 (Spanish)
(301) 670-9292

Lupus Network
230 Ranch Drive
Bridgeport, CT 06606
(203) 372-5795

MARFAN'S SYNDROME

National Marfan Foundation
382 Main Street
Port Washington, NY 11050
(800) 862-7326
(516) 883-8712

MATERNAL AND CHILD HEALTH

ASPO/Lamaze (Psychoprophlaxis In Obstetrics)
1101 Connecticut Avenue, NW
Suite 700
Washington, D.C. 20036
(800) 368-4404
(202) 857-1128

Cesareans/Support Education And Concern
22 Forest Road
Framingham, MA 01701
(508) 877-8266

Depression After Delivery
P.O. Box 1282
Morrisville, PA 19067
(800) 944-4773
(215) 295-3994

National Child Safety Council
Kid Safe Division
P.O. Box 1368
4065 Page Avenue
Jackson, MI 49204-1368
(800) 543-7233

National Maternal And Child Health Clearinghouse
8201 Greensboro Drive
Suite 600
McLean, VA 22102
(703) 821-8955

MEDICATIONS

Drug Information Clearinghouse
Food and Drug Administration
5600 Fishers Lane—HFD8
Rockville, MD 20857
(301) 594-1012

National Information Center For
Orphan Drugs & Rare Diseases
P.O. Box 1133
Washington, D.C. 20013
(800) 336-4797

Nonprescription Drug Manufacturers Association
1150 Connecticut Avenue, NW
Suite 1200
Washington, D.C. 20036
(202) 429-9260

Orphan Products Development
Food and Drug Administration
5600 Fishers Lane
Rockville, MD 20857
(301) 443-2043

MENTAL HEALTH

Association For Children's Mental Health
Woodbrook Village
1705 Coolidge Road
East Lansing, MI 48823
(800) 782-0883
(517) 336-7222

National Alliance For The Mentally Ill
2101 Wilson Boulevard, Suite 302
Arlington, VA 22201
(800) 950-6264

National Clearinghouse On Family
Support And Children's Mental Health
Portland State University
P.O. Box 751
Portland, OR 97207-0751
(800) 628-1696

National Depressive And Manic Depressive
Association
730 North Franklin, Suite 501
Chicago, IL 60610
(800) 826-3632
(312) 642-0049

National Foundation For Depressive Illness
P.O. Box 2257
New York, NY 10116
(800) 248-4344

National Institute Of Mental Health
Information Resources and Inquiries Branch
5600 Fishers Lane
Room 15C-105
Rockville, MD 20857
(301) 443-4515

National Mental Health Association
1021 Prince Street
Alexandria, VA 22314-2971
(800) 433-5959
(703) 684-7722

National Mental Health
Consumer Self-Help Clearinghouse
311 South Juniper Street
Philadelphia, PA 19107
(800) 553-4539
(215) 735-6082

Obsessive Compulsive Foundation
Milford, CT
(203) 878-5669

MENTAL RETARDATION

American Association Of The Mentally Retarded
1719 Kalorama Road, NW
Washington, D.C. 20009
(800) 424-3688
(202) 387-1968

Association For Retarded Citizens
500 East Border
Suite 300
Arlington, TX 76010
(800) 433-5255
(817) 261-6003

MULTIPLE SCLEROSIS

Multiple Sclerosis Foundation
6350 N. Andrews Avenue
Fort Lauderdale, FL 33309
(800) 441-7055

National Multiple Sclerosis Society
733 Third Avenue
New York, NY 10017
(800) 532-7667
(212) 986-3240

MUSCULAR DYSTROPHY

Muscular Dystrophy Association
3300 East Sunrise Drive
Tucson, AZ 85718
(602) 529-2000
New York, NY
(212) 557-8450

NEUROFIBROMATOSIS

National Neurofibromatosis Foundation
141 Fifth Avenue
Suite 7-S
New York, NY 10010
(800) 323-7938
(212) 460-8980

NUTRITION

Consumer Information Center
Consumer Information Catalogue
Pueblo, CO 81009
(719) 948-3334

Food And Nutrition Information Center
National Agricultural Library
Room 304
10301 Baltimore Boulevard
Beltsville, MD 20705
(301) 504-5719

Human Nutrition Information Service, USDA
Federal Building, 6505 Belcrest Road
Hyattsville, MD 20782
(800) 535-4555
(301) 436-8617

National Center For Nutrition And Dietetics
216 W. Jackson Boulevard
Chicago, IL 60606-6995
(800) 366-1655

OCCUPATIONAL SAFETY AND HEALTH

National Institute For Occupational Safety And Health
4676 Columbia Parkway
Cincinnati, OH 45226
(800) 356-4674

ORGAN DONATION AND MARROW TRANSPLANTS

Living Bank International
P.O. Box 6725
Houston, TX 77265
(800) 528-2971

National Marrow Donor Program
3433 Broadway Street, NE, Suite 400
Minneapolis, MN 55413
(800) 654-1247

United Network For Organ Sharing
P.O. Box 13770
Richmond, VA 23225
(800) 243-6667

OSTEOPOROSIS

National Osteoporosis Foundation
1150 17th Street, NW, Suite 500
Washington, D.C. 20036
(800) 223-9994
(202) 223-2226

PAGET'S DISEASE

The Paget Foundation
200 Varick Street
Suite 1004
New York, NY 10014-4810
(800) 237-2438
(212) 229-1582

PAIN

American Chronic Pain Association
P.O. Box 850
Rocklin, CA 95677
(916) 632-0922

National Chronic Pain Outreach
7979 Old Georgetown Road
Suite 100
Bethesda, MD 20814-2429
(301) 652-4948

PARKINSON'S DISEASE

American Parkinson's Disease Association
60 Bay Street, Suite 401
Staten Island, NY 10301
(800) 223-2732
(718) 981-8001

National Parkinson's Foundation
1501 N.W. 9th Avenue
Bob Hope Road
Miami, FL 33136-1494
(800) 327-4545
(305) 547-6666

Parkinson's Disease Foundation
650 W. 168th Street
New York, NY 10032
(800) 457-6676
(212) 923-4700

Parkinson's Educational Program
3900 Birch Street, #105
Newport Beach, CA 92660
(800) 344-7872
(714) 250-2975

POISON CONTROL

American Association of Poison Control Centers
Washington, D.C.
EMERGENCY LINE (202) 625-3333
(202) 784-4666

POLIO

The Polio Society
4200 Wisconsin Avenue, NW, Suite 106273
Washington, D.C. 20016
(301) 897-8180

PRIMARY IMMUNE DEFICIENCY

J. Modell Foundation
Department A, 43 W. 47th Street
New York, NY 10036
(800) 533-3844

PSORIASIS

National Psoriasis Foundation
6600 S.W. 92nd, Suite 300
Portland, OR 97223
(800) 248-0886
(503) 244-7404

The Psoriasis Research Institute
600 Town & Country Center
Palo Alto, CA 94301
(415) 326-1848

RARE DISORDERS

National Information Center For Orphan
Drugs & Rare Diseases
P.O. Box 1133
Washington, D.C. 20013-1133
(800) 336-4797

National Information System & Clearinghouse
(800) 922-9234

National Organization For Rare Disorders, Inc.
P.O. Box 8923
New Fairfield, CT 06812
(800) 447-6673
(203) 746-8825

REHABILITATION

National Rehabilitation Information Center
8455 Colesville Road, Suite 935
Silver Spring, MD 20910
(800) 346-2742

RESPIRATORY

Asthma & Allergy Referral Line
(800) 822-2762

National Jewish Lung Line
(800) 222-5864

REYE'S SYNDROME

National Reye's Syndrome Foundation
426 North Lewis Street
P.O. Box 829
Bryan, OH 43506
(800) 233-7393
(419) 636-2679

SCLERODERMA

Scleroderma Federation
Peabody Office Building
One Newbury Street
Peabody, MA 01960
(800) 422-1113
(508) 535-6600

United Scleroderma Foundation
P.O. Box 399
Watsonville, CA 95077
(800) 722-4673
(408) 728-2202

SCOLIOSIS

National Scoliosis Foundation
72 Mount Auburn Street
Watertown, MA 02172
(617) 926-0397

SEXUALLY TRANSMITTED DISEASES

American Foundation For The Prevention
Of Venereal Disease
799 Broadway, Suite 638
New York, NY 10003
(212) 759-2069

American Social Health Association
P.O. Box 13827
Research Triangle Park, NC 27709
(919) 361-8400

National STD Hotline
(800) 227-8922

National Herpes Hotline
(919) 361-8488

SICKLE CELL DISEASE

National Association For Sickle Cell Disease, Inc.
3345 Wilshire Boulevard, Suite 1106
Los Angeles, CA 90010-1880
(800) 421-8453
(213) 736-5455

SJOGREN'S SYNDROME

Sjogren's Syndrome Foundation
382 Main Street
Port Washington, NY 11050
(516) 767-2866

SLEEP DISORDERS

National Sleep Foundation
122 S. Robertson Boulevard, Third Floor
Los Angeles, CA 90048
(310) 288-0466

SPEECH DISORDERS

American Speech-Language-Hearing Association
10801 Rockville Pike
Rockville, MD 20852
(800) 638-8255
(301) 897-5700

National Center For Stuttering
200 E. 33rd Street, Suite 17C
New York, NY 10016
(800) 221-2483
(212) 532-1460

Stuttering Foundation Of America
P.O. Box 11749
Memphis, TN 38111-0749
(800) 992-9392

SPINA BIFIDA

Spina Bifida Association Of America
4590 MacArthur Boulevard NW
Suite 250
Washington, D.C. 20007-4226
(800) 621-3141
(202) 944-3285

SPINAL CORD INJURY

American Paralysis Association
National Spinal Cord Injury Hot Line
(800) 526-3456

National Coordinating Council On Spinal Cord Injury
801 18th Street, NW
Washington, D.C. 20006
(800) 424-8200

National Spinal Cord Injury Association
600 W. Cummings Park
Suite 2000
Woburn, MA 01801
(800) 962-9629
(617) 935-2722

SPONDYLITIS

Spondylitis Association Of America
P.O. Box 5872
Sherman Oaks, CA 91413
(800) 777-8189

STROKE

National Institute Of Neurological Disorders And Stroke
9000 Rockville Pike
Building 31
Room 8A16
Bethesda, MD 20892
(800) 352-9424

National Stroke Association
8480 East Orchard Road, Suite 1000
Englewood, CO 80111-5015
(800) 787-6537
(303) 771-1700

SUDDEN INFANT DEATH SYNDROME (SIDS)

National Sudden Infant Death Syndrome Resource Center
8201 Greensboro Drive, Suite 600
McLean, VA 22102
(703) 821-8955

Sudden Infant Death Syndrome (SIDS) Alliance
10500 Little Patuxent Parkway, Suite 420
Columbia, MD 21044-3505
(800) 221-7437
(410) 964-8000

TAY-SACHS

National Tay-Sachs And Allied Diseases Association
2001 Beacon Street, Suite 204
Brookline, MA 02146
(617) 277-4463

TINNITUS

American Tinnitus Association
P.O. Box 5
Portland, OR 97207
(503) 248-9985

TOURETTE SYNDROME

Tourette Syndrome Association
42-40 Bell Blvd.
Bayside, NY 11361
(800) 237-0717
(718) 224-2999

TUBEROUS SCLEROSIS

National Tuberous Sclerosis Association
8000 Corporate Drive
Suite 120
Landover, MD 20785
(800) 225-6872
(301) 459-9888

UROLOGIC DISEASE

American Foundation For Urologic Disease
1120 N. Charles Street
Baltimore, MD 21201
(800) 242-2383
(410) 727-2896

VISUAL IMPAIRMENT

American Council Of The Blind
1155 15th Street, NW
Suite 720
Washington, D.C. 20005
(800) 424-8666
(202) 467-5081

American Foundation For The Blind
15 W. 16th Street
New York, NY 10011
(800) 232-5463
(212) 620-2000

Blind Children's Center
4120 Marathon Street
Los Angeles, CA 90029
(800) 222-3566
(800) 222-3567 (in California only)

Library Of Congress "Talking Book" Service
(800) 424-9100

Lighthouse National Center For Vision And Aging
800 2nd Avenue
New York, NY 10017
(800) 334-5497
(212) 808-0077

The National Society To Prevent Blindness
500 E. Remington Road
Schaumburg, IL 60173
(800) 221-3004
(708) 843-2020

Recording For The Blind
(800) 221-4792

National Retinitis Pigmentosa Foundation, Inc.
1401 Mt. Royal Avenue, 4th Floor
Baltimore, MD 21217
(800) 683-5555

The Glaucoma Foundation
310 E. 14th Street
New York, NY 10003
(800) 832-3926
(212) 260-1000

VITILIGO

National Vitiligo Foundation
P.O. Box 6337
Tyler, TX 75711
(903) 534-2925

GENERAL SOURCES

American Academy Of Family Physicians
8880 Ward Parkway
Kansas City, MO 64114-2797
(800) 274-2237
(816) 333-9700

American Academy Of Pediatrics
141 Northwest Point Boulevard
P.O. Box 927
Elk Grove Village, IL 60009
(800) 433-9016

American Board Of Medical Specialties
180 Allen Road, South Building, Suite 300
Atlanta, GA 30328
(800) 776-2378

American College Of Physicians
Independence Mall West
Sixth Street at Race
Philadelphia, PA 19106-1572
(800) 523-1546

American Medical Association
515 North State Street
Chicago, IL 60610
(312) 464-5000

American Osteopathic Association
42 East Ontario
Chicago, IL 60611
(800) 621-1773
(312) 280-5800

American Red Cross
431 18th Street, N.W.
Washington, D.C. 20006
(202) 737-8300

Consumer Information Center
Consumer Information Catalogue
Pueblo, CO 81009
(719) 948-3334

National Foundation For Infectious Diseases
4733 Bethesda Avenue, Suite 750
Bethesda, MD 20814
(301) 656-0003

National Vaccine Information Center
512 West Maple Avenue, Suite 206
Vienna, VA 22180
(703) 938-3783

National Women's Health Resource Center
2440 M Street, NW, Suite 325
Washington, D.C. 20037
(202) 293-6045

Office of Disease Prevention And Health Promotion
National Health Information Center
P.O. Box 1133
Washington, D.C. 20013-1133
(800) 336-4797
(301) 565-4020

STATE INSURANCE OFFICES

ALABAMA

Alabama Insurance Department
135 South Union Street
Montgomery, Alabama 36130-3315
(205) 269-3550

ALASKA

Alaska Insurance Department
800 East Dimond Boulevard, Suite 560
Anchorage, Alaska 99515
(907) 349-1230

ARIZONA

Arizona Insurance Department
2910 North 44th Street, Suite 210
Phoenix, Arizona 85018
(602) 912-8400; (602) 912-8444

ARKANSAS

Arkansas Insurance Department
400 University Tower Building
Little Rock, Arkansas 72204
(501) 686-2945

CALIFORNIA

California Insurance Department
300 South Spring Street
Los Angeles, California 90013
(213) 897-8921

COLORADO

Colorado Insurance Department
1560 Broadway
Suite 850
Denver, Colorado 80202
(303) 894-7499

CONNECTICUT

Connecticut Insurance Department
P.O. Box 816
Hartford, Connecticut 06142-0816
(203) 297-3800

DELAWARE

Delaware Insurance Department
841 Silver Lake Boulevard
Dover, Delaware 19901
(302) 739-4251

DISTRICT OF COLOMBIA

District of Colombia
613 G Street, N.W.
Room 603
Washington, D.C. 20001-7200
(202) 727-8017

FLORIDA

Florida Insurance Department
200 East Gaines Street
Tallahassee, Florida 32399-0300
(904) 922-3100

GEORGIA

Georgia Insurance Department
2 Martin Luther King, Jr., Drive
7th Floor Floyd Building
Atlanta, Georgia 30334
(404) 656-2056

HAWAII

Hawaii Insurance Department
1010 Richards Street
5th floor
Honolulu, Hawaii 96813
(808) 586-2790

IDAHO

Idaho Insurance Department
700 West State Street
Boise, Idaho 83720
(208) 334-4350

ILLINOIS

Illinois Insurance Department
320 West Washington Street
Springfield, Illinois 62767
(217) 782-4515

INDIANA

Indiana Insurance Department
311 West Washington Street
Suite 300
Indianapolis, Indiana 46204
(317) 232-2385

IOWA

Iowa Insurance Division
Lucas State Office Building
Des Moines, Iowa
(515) 281-5705

KANSAS

Kansas Insurance Department
420 S.W. 9th Street
Topeka, Kansas 66612-1678
(913) 296-3071

KENTUCKY

Kentucky Insurance Department
P.O. 517
Frankfort, Kentucky 40602
(502) 564-3630

LOUISIANA

Louisiana Insurance Department
P.O. Box 94214
Baton Rouge, Louisiana 70804-9214
(504) 342-5900

MAINE

Maine Insurance Department
State House
Station 34
Augusta, Maine 04333
(207) 582-8707

MARYLAND

Maryland Insurance Department
501 St. Paul Place
Baltimore, Maryland 21202
(410) 333-2792

MASSACHUSETTS

Massachusetts Insurance Department
280 Friend Street
Boston, Massachusetts 02114
(617) 727-7189

MICHIGAN

Michigan Insurance Department
P.O. Box 30220
Lansing, Michigan 48909
(517) 373-0220

MINNESOTA

Minnesota Insurance Department
133 East 7th Street
St. Paul, Minnesota 55101
(612) 296-4026

MISSISSIPPI

Mississippi Insurance Department
P.O. Box 79
Jackson, Mississippi 39205
(601) 359-3569

MISSOURI

Missouri Insurance Department
P.O. Box 690
Jefferson City, Missouri 65102
(314) 751-2640

MONTANA

Montana Insurance Department
P.O. Box 4009
Helena, Montana 59604-4009
(406) 444-2040

NEBRASKA

Nebraska Insurance Department
941 O Street, Suite 400
Lincoln, Nebraska 68508
(402) 471-2201

NEVADA

Nevada Insurance Department
1665 Hot Springs Road, Suite 152
Carson City, Nevada 89710
(702) 687-4270

NEW HAMPSHIRE

New Hampshire Insurance Department
169 Manchester Street
Concord, New Hampshire 03301
(603) 271-2261

NEW JERSEY

New Jersey Insurance Department
20 West State Street, CN 329
Trenton, New Jersey 08625
(609) 292-4757

NEW MEXICO

New Mexico Insurance Department
P.O. Drawer 1269
Pera Building
Santa Fe, New Mexico 87504-1269
(505) 827-4500

NEW YORK

New York Insurance Department
160 West Broadway
New York, New York 10013-3393
(212) 602-0203

NORTH CAROLINA

North Carolina Insurance Department
P.O. Box 26387
Raleigh, North Carolina 27611
(919) 733-2004

NORTH DAKOTA

North Dakota Insurance Department
600 East Boulevard Avenue
5th Floor
Bismarck, North Dakota 58505
(701) 224-2440

OHIO

Ohio Insurance Department
2100 Stella Court
Columbus, Ohio 43266-0566
(614) 644-2673

OKLAHOMA

Oklahoma Insurance Department
P.O. Box 53408
Oklahoma City, Oklahoma 73152-3408
(405) 521-2828

OREGON

Oregon Insurance Department
440-2 Labor Industry Building
Salem, Oregon 97310
(503) 378-4636

PENNSYLVANIA

Pennsylvania Insurance Department
1321 Strawberry Square
Harrisburg, Pennsylvania 17120-0027
(717) 787-2317

RHODE ISLAND

Rhode Island Insurance Department
233 Richard Street, Suite 233
Providence, Rhode Island 02903-4233
(410) 277-2223

SOUTH CAROLINA

South Carolina Insurance Department
P.O. Box 100105
Columbia, South Carolina 29202
(803) 737-6140

SOUTH DAKOTA

South Dakota Insurance Department
500 East Capitol
Pierre, South Dakota 57501-5070
(605) 773-3563

TENNESSEE

Tennessee Insurance Department
500 James Robertson Parkway
4th Floor
Nashville, Tennessee 37243-0582
(615) 741-4955

TEXAS

Texas Insurance Department
P.O. Box 149104
Austin, Texas 78714-9104
(512) 463-6169

UTAH

Utah Insurance Department
State Office Building
Room 3110
Salt Lake City, Utah 84114
(801) 538-3800

VERMONT

Vermont Insurance Department
89 Main Street
Drawer 20
Montpelier, Vermont 05620-3101
(802) 828-3301

VIRGINIA

Virginia Insurance Department
P.O. Box 1157
Richmond, Virginia 23209-1157
(804) 371-9691

WASHINGTON

Washington Insurance Department
P.O. Box 40255
Olympia, Washington 98504-0255
(206) 753-7300

WEST VIRGINIA

West Virginia Insurance Department
2019 Washington Street, East
Charleston, West Virginia 25305
(304) 558-3386

WISCONSIN

Wisconsin Insurance Department
P.O. Box 7873
Madison, Wisconsin 53707
(608) 266-0103

WYOMING

Wyoming Insurance Department
122 West 25th Street
Cheyenne, Wyoming 82002
(307) 777-7401

Believe It Or Not, It's Free

Contrary to conventional wisdom, there actually sometimes is a free lunch in life. However, in order to "qualify" for that free lunch, at least when it comes to health care, you really must be in need. What follows is a summary of places to look for free or greatly reduced prices on health care. In most cases, eligibility is based on need and need is usually determined by government-set standards on income and poverty levels.

One thing always to keep in mind is that there are resources out there if you really need them and are willing to look for them. Your local library is a great first step when seeking information specific to your city, county and state. For example, there are a number of grants that are administered to help people in need, many with a focus on health concerns. Some of these grants are given to individuals based solely on where they live. So, begin your search by checking the reference section of your library and reviewing available grants.

Another potential source for help in meeting special or emergency health needs is your employer. Many employers, especially large corporations, offer special assistance to employees with special health care needs (this courtesy usually extends to immediate family members). Your personnel office or human resources department should be able to give you more information.

Do you have school age children? The Parent Teachers Association (PTA) at your child's school may have programs designed to help families meet basic health care needs. In many communities, the PTA operates clinics for checkups and immunizations. In some communities, the PTA is even involved in dental clinics. Finally, local PTA chapters are often available to help a family in need purchase corrective glasses for children.

Additionally, there are a number of civic organizations whose mission is to help people in the community. These groups often earmark specific funds for health and medical needs and include the Elks, Kiwanis and Rotary clubs. To contact the local chapter of one of these clubs in your community, check the yellow pages of your phone book. If you can't find a local listing, call your chamber of commerce, which should be able to refer you to the closest club.

Here are some additional resources offering help on a national basis.

HOSPITAL AND NURSING HOME CARE

Hill-Burton Program
(800) 638-0742
In Maryland, (800) 492-0359

This federal government program offers free or low-cost health care to people who cannot afford to pay. Eligibility is based on income: your income must fall within the Poverty Guidelines determined by the Department of Health and Human Services. At some facilities, care may still be offered to those with incomes up to twice the amount dictated by the Poverty Guidelines.

Hill-Burton assistance only covers facility charges, not physician fees. To identify facilities in your area that offer free care through Hill-Burton, call the telephone number listed above. Once the facilities are identified, you can begin steps necessary to obtain care: first, securing your eligibility and then determining what care is available to you.

Facilities participating in the program include hospitals and nursing homes. These facilities are required to offer a certain amount of free care each year. Once the care level is achieved, the free benefit is no longer available. As a result, care facilities in your area that participate in the program must be further identified as still needing to meet their "free" care requirement for the year.

EYE AND VISION CARE

Lions Club
Foundation (708) 681-8800
International (708) 571-5466
Eye Bank (800) 933-3937

The Lions Club is a civic organization dedicated to protecting sight, preventing blindness and facilitating eye transplantation.

One program that is most helpful and easily accessible on a local level is "Sight First." This program fights blindness, supports research and, on a more personal level, will provide funds for eye exams and corrective lenses for needy individuals.

To find out more about this service, call your local chapter of the Lions Club. If you are unable to find a local listing, call your chamber of commerce for the telephone numbers of the Lions Club in your area. These local clubs are most interested in working to protect the sight of needy individuals.

MUSCULAR AND ORTHOPEDIC CARE FOR CHILDREN

Shriners Hospitals
(800) 237-5055
In Florida, (800) 282-9161

The Shriners support hospital care for children under age 18 who have muscular or orthopedic problems, or who are burn victims. The Shriners have a network of twenty-two hospitals, which offer care free of charge to qualified patients. Call the hotline numbers listed above to discuss your specific situation.

CANCER TREATMENT

National Cancer Institute's Information Service
(800) 422-6237

This service offers information on current therapies. This is an excellent source of information regarding current clinical trials of experimental treatments. Individuals who are chosen to participate in such trials receive treatment at no charge.

HEARING SERVICES

Hear Now
(800) 648-4327

This organization works to make hearing aids, cochlear implants and other hearing services available to those with limited financial resources. To receive assistance, call the telephone number listed above for an application.

AFTERWORD

We hope you've found the information in this book helpful. If you haven't already begun using it to reduce your health care costs, give one of our suggestions a try today. See how it can reduce your medical expenses and improve the quality of the care you receive. The sooner all of us begin following these recommendations, the sooner we can collectively begin to improve our health care system, making it work better for everyone.

We would also like to hear from you. Please write us at the address below, and tell us how you've saved money in obtaining medical services. We plan to use some of this feedback in future editions of this book. If we include your suggestions (with your name, if you'd like), we'll send you a free copy of the revised book, along with a sincere thank you for helping all of us get more for our health care dollar.

Please write to us in care of:

Ulysses Press
P.O. Box 3440
Berkeley, CA 94703-3440

We wish you good luck—and good health.

GLOSSARY

Some Common Health Care Terms & What They Mean

Throughout this book, we've referred to terms commonly used in the health care industry, and which often cause more confusion than clarity. Here are definitions that will help guide you through the maze of jargon and medicalese.

Benefit period: A predetermined length of time during which a new deductible applies and health insurance benefits are paid, such as a calendar year or for the length of the contract.

Catastrophic coverage: Health insurance that provides protection specifically against major illness and injury. It typically has a high maximum benefit, often up to $1 million, and may cover health care costs (e.g., for doctors, hospital, medications) not covered by a base insurance plan.

COBRA: The Consolidated Omnibus Budget Reconciliation Act, a law passed by Congress, that permits a covered employee and dependents to extend their health coverage after the covered employee leaves his or her job and its employee health plan.

Co-insurance: Also called "co-payment," this is the percentage of your medical bills for which you are responsible. In a typical policy, you will pay 20 percent of the charges, and the insurance company will cover the remaining 80 percent (once you have met your deductible).

Co-payment: See "co-insurance."

Deductible: The amount of health care expenses you are responsible for paying each benefit period out-of-pocket before the insurance company starts covering any of your costs. Thus, if you have a $250 annual deductible, you alone must pay the first $250 of your medical bills in full each year before your insurance will pay any percentage.

Fee-for-service: In this traditional type of coverage, you are free to choose your own doctor and your insurance company pays the doctor or hospital for each service that is rendered.

Generic: Drugs that are basically chemically identical to brand-name (or proprietary) medications, and are approved for marketing once the original patent of the proprietary drug has expired. These generic products are marketed under the name attached to them in their early development, and tend to be less expensive than their brand-name counterparts (i.e., ibuprofen is the generic drug, while Motrin is a name brand).

Health maintenance organization (HMO): An organization providing all health care services to its enrolled participants at a fixed, agreed-upon fee.

Individual practice association (IPA): A form of practice in which doctors sign contracts to provide treatment for subscribers of organizations like HMOs. These physicians do not have exclusive contracts with these organizations, however, and thus may also treat patients who are not HMO members.

Inpatient: Care provided to patients staying overnight at a facility like a hospital.

Lifetime maximum benefit: The total amount that an insurance policy will pay for given benefits. It is often expressed in a dollar amount (e.g., $1 million coverage over a lifetime). Once the maximum is reached, no further payment will be made by the insurer ever.

Major medical: Health coverage for a major illness or injury (See "catastrophic illness").

Managed care: A health care system (like an HMO) that provides comprehensive services to subscribers, while incorporating a financial incentive for using the services of that system exclusively. These programs generally have guidelines for receiving care and for ensuring the quality of that treatment.

Medicaid: Supplemental health care programs operated by each of the 50 states, and made available to people with limited resources, without regard to their age.

Medigap: Private insurance policies designed to supplement the coverage provided by Medicare. Also referred to as "Medicare supplemental insurance."

Out-of-pocket: The portion of medical expenses that must be paid by the policyholder that are not reimbursed the insurance company. These expenses generally include the "deductible" and "co-payment" for which the policyholder is responsible.

Outpatient: Medical care provided to individuals outside of a traditional hospital setting when no overnight stay is required, such as in a doctor's office, a clinic, or other medical facility, including a hospital's own outpatient center.

Over-the-counter drugs: Medications that can be purchased without a physician's prescription (also called nonprescription drugs).

Pre-existing conditions: Diseases or disorders that a person already has been treated for before buying a health insurance policy, and which the insurance company may not cover, at least not until a lengthy waiting period has passed.

Preferred Provider Organization (PPO): A group of doctors (or hospitals) that provides health care to subscribers of a medical insurance plan, generally at reduced costs.

Premium: The monthly, quarterly, semi-annual or annual fee paid for insurance coverage. In some plans, the employer pays part of the premium and the employee pays the remainder; sometimes, the premium is completely covered by the employer.

Prescription drugs: Medications that can only be obtained with a prescription written by a physician.

Skilled nursing facility: A site certified by Medicare (and/or Medicaid) to offer daily nursing care that is provided by trained medical staff.

Stop loss provision: A clause in an insurance contract that sets a ceiling on the amount of co-insurance for which a policyholder is responsible. It is often part of a major medical insurance policy.

Subscriber: A purchaser of, or an enrollee in, an insurance policy or an HMO.

Usual and customary: The typical fees charged by doctors in a community for a given procedure as determined by an insurance company. In order to control costs, insurance companies often will not reimburse patients for bills over this amount, even if the doctor's charges are higher.

REFERENCES

Bernstein S.J., Hilborne L.H., Leape L.L., Fiske M.E., Park R.E., Kamberg C.J., Brook R.H. "The Appropriateness of Use of Coronary Angiography in New York State." *JAMA* 26 (1993): 766–769.

Braveman P., Geraldine O., Miller M.G., Reiter R., Egerte S. "Adverse Outcomes and Lack of Health Insurance Among Newborns in an Eight-County Area of California, 1982 to 1986." *New England Journal of Medicine* 321 (1989): 508–513.

Bueschling D.P., Jablonowski A., Vesta E., Ditts W., Runge C., Lund J., Porter R. "Inappropriate Emergency Department Visits." *Annals of Emergency Medicine* 14 (1985): 672–676.

Chassin M.R., Brook R.H., Park R.E., Keesey J., Fink A., Kosecoff J., Kahn K., Merrick N., Solomon D.H. "Variations in the Use of Medical and Surgical Services by the Medicare Population." *New England Journal of Medicine* 314 (1986): 285–290.

Chassin M.R., Kosecoff J., Park R.E., Winslow C.M., Kahn K.L., Merrick N.J., Keesey J., Fink A., Solomon D.H., Brook R.H. "Does Inappropriate Use Explain Geographic Variations in the Use of Health Care Services: A Study of Three Procedures." *JAMA* 258 (1987): 2533–2537.

Chu A., Lavoie V., McCarthy E.G. "Second Opinion Programs: Continued Savings From Nonconfirmed Surgeries." *Employee Benefits Journal.* (September 1992): 35–40.

Dyckman Z. "Physician cost experience under private health insurance programs." *Health Care Financing Review* 13 (1992): 85–96.

Hadley J., Steinberg E.P., Feder J. "Comparison of Uninsured and Privately Insured Hospital Patients: Condition on Admission, Resource Use, and Outcome." *JAMA* 265 (1991): 374–379.

Hannan E.L., O'Donnell J.F., Kilburn H., Bernard H.R., Yazici A. "Investigation of the Relationship Between Volume and Mortality for Surgical Procedures Performed in New York State Hospitals." *JAMA* 262 (1989): 503–510.

Hilborne L.H., Leape L.L., Bernstein S.J., Park R.E., Fiske M.E., Kamberg C.J., Roth C.P., Brook R.H. "The Appropriateness of Use of Percutaneous Transluminal Coronary Angioplasty in New York State." *JAMA* 269 (1993): 761–765.

Hillman B.J., Joseph C.A., Mabry M.R., Sunshine J.H., Kennedy S.D., Noether M. "Frequency and Costs of Diagnostic Imaging in Office Practice—A Comparison of Self-Referring and Radiologist-Referring Physicians." *New England Journal of Medicine* 323 (1990): 1604–1608.

Kaplan E.B., Sheiner L.B., Boeckmann A.J., Roizen M.F., Beal S.L., Cohen S.N., Nicoll C.D. "The Usefulness of Preoperative Laboratory Screening." *JAMA* 253 (1985): 3576–3581.

Kitz D.S., Slusarz-Ladden C., Lecky J.H. "Hospital Resources Used for Inpatient and Ambulatory Surgery." *Anesthesiology* 69 (1988): 383–386.

Leape L.L., Hilborne L.H., Park R.E., Bernstein S.J., Kamberg C.J., Sherwood M., Brook R.H. "The Appropriateness of Use of Coronary Artery Bypass Graft Surgery in New York State." *JAMA* 269 (1993): 753–760.

Leary W.E. "Outpatient Surgery on the Rise; Regulation Doesn't Keep Pace." *New York Times.* July 1, 1992

Levit K.R., Cowan C.A. "Business, Households, and Governments: Health Care Costs, 1990." *Health Care Financing Review* 13 (1991): 83–93.

Levit K.R., Lazenby H.C., Cowan C.A., Letsch S.W. "National Health Expenditures, 1990." *Health Care Financing Review* 13 (1991): 29–54.

LoGerfo J.P., Efird R.A., Diehr P.K., Richardson W.C. "Rates of Surgical Care in Prepaid Group Practices and the Independent Setting: What are the Reasons for the Differences?" *Medical Care* 17 (1979): 1–7.

Lundberg G. Editorial. *JAMA* 249 (1983): 639.

Mozes B., Schiff E., Modan B. "Factors Affecting Inappropriate Hospital Stay." *Quality Assurance in Health Care* 3 (1991): 211–217.

Nagurney J.T., Braham R.L., Reader G.G.. "Physician Awareness of Economic Factors in Clinical Decision-Making." *Medical Care* 17 (1979): 727–736.

Reff D., DelGiudice G., Aisen P., Winters S., Gorlin R. "Medical Cost Containment: A Daily Patient Log Sheet to Reduce Unnecessary Hospitalization." *The Mount Sinai Journal of Medicine* 54 (1987): 496–499.

Safavi K.T., Hayward R.A. "Choosing between Apples and Apples: Physicians' Choices of Prescription Drugs That Have Similar Side Effects and Efficacies." *Journal of General Internal Medicine* 7 (1992): 32–37.

Selker H.P., Beshansky J.R., Paulker S.G., Kassirer J.P. "The Epidemiology of Delays in a Teaching Hospital: The Development and Use of a Tool that Detects Unnecessary Hospital Days." *Medical Care* 27 (1989): 112–122.

Siu A.L., Sonnenberg F.A., Manning W.G., Goldberg G.A., Bloomfield E.S., Newhouse J.P., Brook R.H. "Inappropriate Use of Hospitals in a Randomized Trial of Health Insurance Plans." *New England Journal of Medicine* 315 (1986): 1259–1266.

Tierney W.M., Miller M.E., McDonald C.J. "The Effect on Test Ordering of Informing Physicians of the Charges for Outpatient Diagnostic Tests." *New England Journal of Medicine* 322 (1990): 1499–1504.

Wallack S.S. "Managed Care: Practice, Pitfalls, and Potential." *Health Care Financing Review* (1991 [supp]): 27–34.

Welch W.P., Miller M.E., Welch H.G., Fisher E.S., Wennberg J.E. "Geographic Variation in Expenditures for Physicians' Services in the United States." *New England Journal of Medicine* 328 (1993): 621–627.

Report of the U.S. Preventive Services Task Force. Guide to Clinical Preventive Services: an Assessment of the Effectiveness of 169 Interventions. Baltimore, Maryland: William and Wilkins; 1989.

"Socioeconomic Characteristics of Medical Practice." *American Medical Association* (1992).

U.S. Department of Health and Human Services, Health Care Financing Administration. *The Medicare 1993 Handbook.* Publication No. HCFA 10050.

INDEX

About the Authors

Dr. Art Ulene has been known to television viewers over the past two decades through his medical reports on the NBC "Today Show" and the ABC "HOME Show." Additionally, he is the author of numerous books and the producer of several video and audio programs. He lives in Los Angeles.

Dr. Ulene's co-author is his daughter, Dr. Val Ulene, also a medical doctor. In addition to the medical degree which she received from Columbia University, Dr. Val Ulene holds a master's degree in public health. She lives in New York City.

OTHER BOOKS BY DR. ART ULENE AND DR. VAL ULENE:

Count Out Cholesterol......................................$12.95

> Complete with counter and detailed dietary
> plan, this companion resource to the cook-
> book shows how to design a cholesterol-low-
> ering program that's right for you.

Count Out Cholesterol Cookbook....................$14.95

> A companion guide to *Count Out Cholesterol*,
> this book shows you how to bring your cho-
> lesterol levels down with the help of 250
> gourmet recipes.

The Vitamin Strategy......................................$11.95

> A game plan for good health, this book helps
> readers design a vitamin and mineral pro-
> gram tailored to their individual needs.

Discovery Play...$9.95

> By Dr. Art Ulene and Dr. Steven Shelov, this
> book guides readers through the first eighteen
> months of parenting with a special emphasis
> on nurturing self-esteem.

*To order these or other Ulysses Press books call 800-
377-2542 or write to Ulysses Press P.O. Box 3440,
Berkeley, CA 94703-3440. **All retail orders are
shipped free of charge.** California residents must
include sales tax. Allow two to three weeks for delivery.*